PREGNANCY AND GESTATION

in Chinese Classical Texts

Monkey Press is named after the Monkey King in The Journey to the West, the 16th century novel by Wu Chengen. Monkey blends skill, initiative and wisdom with the spirit of freedom, irreverence and mischief.

ALSO PUBLISHED BY MONKEY PRESS:
The Way of Heaven: Neijing Suwen chapters 1 and 2
The Secret Treatise of the Spiritual Orchid: Suwen chapter 8
The Seven Emotions
The Eight Extraordinary Meridians
The Extraordinary Fu
Essence Spirit Blood and Qi
The Lung
The Kidneys
Spleen and Stomach
The Heart in Lingshu chapter 8
The Liver
Heart Master Triple Heater
A Study of Qi
Yin Yang in Classical Texts
The Essential Woman

PREGNANCY AND GESTATION
in Chinese Classical Texts

Elisabeth Rochat de la Vallée

MONKEY PRESS

© Monkey Press 2007

PREGNANCY AND GESTATION

Elisabeth Rochat de la Vallée

ISBN 978 1 872468 38 9

www.monkeypress.net
monkey.press@virgin.net

Text Editor: Caroline Root
Production and Design: Sandra Hill
Cover image: Court Women, Tang Dynasty

Printed on recycled paper by
Biddles Ltd, Kings Lynn, Norfolk

CONTENTS

FOREWORD

This new book by Elisabeth Rochat de la Vallée presents the various transformations which occur within the mother and developing baby during pregnancy. Beginning with Suwen chapter 1, which describes the unfolding of female fertility, Elisabeth then looks at descriptions of the pulses during pregnancy.

A month-by-month description of pregnancy is given drawing specifically on the Zhubing Yuanhou Lun, the Mawangdui Manuscript and Sun Simiao. Two later texts considered, the Qipolun and the Luxingjing, are particularly interesting because they present alternative and more unusual images of the developing fetus, and speak of the presence of the spirits (*hun*, *po* and *shen*) in the fetus.

These ancient teachings are still valuable today for our understanding of the transformations of blood and *qi* which take place during the ten months of a pregnancy. The material will be of great help to those working with pregnant women or simply interested in the process of pregnancy. Together with its companion volume, The Essential Woman, Elisabeth Rochat has given us two indispensable guides to the classical Chinese perception of women's health and fertility.The explanations and insights offered will be of immense help to all those considering and treating women with their 'equal but different' nature.

Translations from the original Chinese are made by

Elisabeth unless otherwise stated. *Qi* is used in the plural to indicate more clearly its meaning in these texts. We include Chinese characters throughout for clarity and understanding, and recommend the use of Dr. S. L. Wieger's Chinese Characters (Dover Language Books) for further analysis.

Caroline Root, December 2007

INTRODUCTION

The subject of this seminar is pregnancy and all the changes and transformations which mother and growing baby go through. I want to start by reminding you of the importance of Suwen chapter 1 where there is a full presentation of a woman's fertility (cf: The Essential Woman: Female Health and Fertility in Chinese Classical Texts, Monkey Press, 2007). We will then look briefly at some texts which describe the pulses of pregnant women, and afterwards will consider other ancient, non-medical texts, such as Huainanzi chapter 7 (2nd century BCE), which give ideas about the development of the fetus. We will also follow the changing physiology of the pregnant woman and her baby as they are described in three texts: the Zhubing Yuanhou Lun, which is a text from the early 7th century CE, the Mawangdui Manuscript from the 2nd century BCE, and Sun Simiao (581-682 CE). These three texts have a lot in common.

We will then look at two other texts, the Qipolun and the Luxinjing, which are of later composition and not really medical. They are interesting because they present other images of the development of the fetus and speak in a non-medical way, taking into account the *hun* (魂) and *po* (魄) souls, and offering various possibilities for the time of their appearance in the fetus.

Our aim is to identify which ideas from these various ancient teachings are still helpful today in our understanding of the transformations of blood and *qi* during the ten months of a pregnancy.

SUWEN CHAPTER 1

In Suwen chapter 1 it says:

'[In a woman of] two times seven years, fertility (*tian gui* 天 癸) arrives. *Ren mai* (任 脈) functions fully while the powerful *chong mai* (衝 脈) rises in power (*sheng* 盛). The menses flow downwards in their time and she has children (*you zi* 有 子).'

This passage shows the great importance of *ren* and *chong mai*, not only for the physiology of women in general but also very specifically for and during pregnancy. The *chong mai* (衝 脈) is the sea of blood and it rules the circulation of blood. The *ren mai* (任 脈) is the source of *yin* within the body, supporting all the *yin* aspects of the physiology and therefore the quality of the blood which is available. So *ren* and *chong mai* play specific roles in the physiology of a woman because of the particular way blood is used in her body, which is different from the way it is used in a man.

When a woman is pregnant a change takes place in the circulation of her blood because it no longer gathers in the uterus waiting to be expelled during menstruation.

Instead, the blood is attracted downwards in order to nourish the embryo and fetus. It is the specific activity of the *chong mai* to ensure a regular movement of blood descending into the uterus for this purpose. The *ren mai* ensures that there is a sufficient quantity of blood and essences for use in the woman's body and for the fetus as it develops.

PULSES IN PREGNANCY

At the very beginning of gestation changes in the pattern of the circulation of the blood and *qi* can be felt on the pulses. This is normal since the pulses are simply the reflection of the state, movement and balance of the blood and *qi* inside the body. Since there is a change in the movement of blood and *qi* due to the pregnancy, that has to be perceptible on the pulses. Of course the problem is that things are not so simple, and there are several possible approaches.

Suwen chapter 40 asks:

"'How do we know when a woman is pregnant?"
Qi Bo replied: "The body is sick (*bing* 病) but the pulses have no perversion (*wu xie mai* 無 邪 脈)."'

We have to understand that the woman will present certain signs in her body which may at first be considered pathological. For instance, the first thing is that menstruation ceases. However, even if she no longer menstruates but does not have pulses which correspond to a case of amenorrhoea, or if she has early morning sickness and feels tired, there may still be no indication that she is pregnant at the level of the pulses.

The classical texts do not say exactly when it is possible to first detect pregnancy, but I think we need at least a month. A commentator on the Neijing, Ma Shi from the 16th century, said: 'In the first month of pregnancy, the essences of *yin* and *yang* are not yet transformed.'

In the second month, he continued, the essences and *qi* change, and the *qi* move upwards and cause morning sickness. In the third and fourth months the morning sickness stops and the pulses are slippery and fast. In the fifth and sixth months there is a stabilization of the form of the fetus. At this time you can also detect whether the woman is expecting a boy or a girl. We will look at this idea in detail later on.

One of the most basic texts on this subject is Suwen chapter 7:

'When the *yin* pulse beats strongly and the *yang* pulse gives the feeling of taking another direction (*yin bo yang bie* 陰 搏 陽 別), it is a sign of pregnancy.'

The *yin* pulse is the distal pulse and the *yang* pulse is the proximal pulse. But you could also say that the *yin* pulses are the deep pulses and the *yang* pulses the superficial pulses. The problem is that in Suwen chapter 7 it is nearly impossible to say which is which. In other texts the usual interpretation is that the *yin* pulse represents the *shao yin* (少 陰), therefore the kidneys and the heart, and the *yang* pulses show the *yang*. When there are these differences between the *yin* and the *yang* there is a pregnancy. The underlying meaning is that there is a strength in the blood indicating that it is gathering. The *yin* movement in the body is strong because there needs to be a process of gathering, concentrating and storing inside. This *yin* movement is strong while the *yang* is separating and is less strong proportionally than the *yin*. The feeling under the fingers when reading the pulses is that the *yang* seems to be going sideways and not staying in a straight circulation. This is a very simple approach. However, at the beginning of a pregnancy it is necessary for the *yin* to be very strong in order to start something. This is the same thing as is described in Zhuangzi chapter 22:

'Man's life is a coming-together of breath (*qi* 氣). If it comes together (*ju* 聚), there is life; if it scatters (*san* 散), there is death.' (Translation by Burton Watson)

Even if Zhuangzi was not thinking of an embryo when he was writing the text this is exactly the same process as for any new life.

Another text which is more precise about the pulses of a pregnant woman is Suwen chapter 18:

'In a woman when the pulse of the *shao yin* of the hand (or foot according to other versions) beats strongly, it is a sign of pregnancy.'

The commentators give three different explanations for this passage. First, it is the pulse felt on the *shao yin* of the hand meridian, the heart, at the level of *shen men* (神 門, Heart 7). This pulse is said to feel big, like a pea, striking and beating. Since in Chinese the same character is used for both pulse and vital circulations (*mai* 脈), we can understand that the text does not necessarily refer only to a 'pulse', but to the quality of blood and *qi* inside the circulation of the heart meridian. The power of the blood in the heart meridian, is the sign of the pregnancy.

A second interpretation is that the 'pulse' here refers to the pulse which you feel in the heart position of the radial pulse, thus implying there is a strong pulse in the heart position. We can understand that the heart and the hand *shao yin* may be implied because the other meridian of the heart (*xin zhu* 心 主, *jue yin* of hand) masters the blood and the blood's circulation. (cf: The Double Aspect of the Heart; Monkey Press 2008). So in this case there is a specific power in the blood. The blood is full and it is possible to see this in the heart pulse or the hand *shao yin* if we think that the beginning of a new life is a question of essences and perhaps spirits.

Therefore even at the level of *shen men*, Heart 7, we can recognise that the woman is pregnant.

Sticking with the physical signs, it is the richness of the blood in the body of the woman which is the indicator, and we perceive that in the heart. Maybe there is even something else which can be felt at the level of the spirits of the heart, but that is a more personal interpretation where the essences are presented as the coming together of two spirits:

'The embrace of two spirits (*er shen* 二 神), by this conjunction (*he* 合), gives form to a body (*cheng xing* 成 形). Always that which comes first in the personal life is called the essences (*jing* 精).' Lingshu chapter 30

According to some commentaries you can even say that if the pulse is more superficial at the level of the hand *tai yang*, the small intestine, it is a boy. But we will come back to this question of boy versus girl later on.

A third interpretation is that it is the pulse felt on the *shao yin* of the foot, the kidney meridian. Rather than understand that it is the pulse of the *shao yin* on the foot (on the ankle artery at the point Kidney 3), the commentators prefer the location of the kidneys on the radial pulses on both sides (*yin* and *yang*) at the proximal pulse. A strong beating in these places is the sign of a pregnancy because it is the sign of the powerful activity of the kidneys which is required at the beginning of a pregnancy. In the beginning, concentration and keeping in the depths are the main thing. It is the precise quality of the kidneys to be able to do this concentrating and keeping in the depths of the essences. It would therefore be normal to feel their dominance on the pulses at this time.

PULSES IN THE ZHUBING YUANHOU LUN

The Zhubing Yuanhou Lun means The Treatise on the Origin and Symptoms of all Disease. It is a book dating from the Sui Dynasty and published in 610 CE, and is a compilation of different writings compiled by Chao Yuan-fang. China had been in great turmoil for some time from the 4th and 5th centuries onwards. There had been many wars and divisions but unity was restored by the Sui Dynasty (589-618 CE) which had a very strong Emperor. In the chaos of the previous era many texts had been lost, but the newly established dynasty tried to reorganize things, and under imperial orders the best texts in every field of knowledge were collected together. The person in charge of collecting and editing medical texts put together the Zhubing Yuanhou Lun. It is a book which was used as a text book for several centuries in medical schools in China. It was composed as a text book. It is not the work of a genius! It is an impersonal work, unlike Sun Simiao or the Shanghan Lun. Sometimes this is good because it means the compiler collected a variety of different but equally interesting texts.

In the Zhubing Yuanhou Lun there is a chapter devoted to pregnancy. It starts with the pulses and recalls quotations from the classics, specifically Suwen chapter 7 where it says that the *yin* beats strongly and the *yang* is different or separating a little:

'When the *yin* pulse beats strongly and the *yang* pulse gives the feeling of taking another direction.'

It adds the explanation that this is a sign that blood and *qi* are in an harmonious composition, but the *yang* displays itself while the *yin* is under transformation. This is the same movement which we feel in the pulses as described in Suwen chapter 7. After this the text of the Zhubing Yuanhou Lun comes to the idea presented in Suwen chapter 18 about the *shao yin*, which we saw above:

'When in a woman the pulse of the *shao yin* of the hand (or foot) beats strongly, it is a sign of pregnancy.'

It says that the *shao yin* is the pulse of the *mai* of the heart because the heart masters the blood circulation. However, immediately afterwards the text speaks about the kidneys:

'The kidneys are called the gate of the uterus (*bao men* 胞門), the door of the child (*zi hu* 子戶). The pulse (*mai* 脈) of the kidneys is full in the proximal position of the pulses, and if on palpation the pulse comes continually without interruption, this is a sign that the woman is pregnant.'

So the *mai* or the pulse of the kidneys is full in the proximal position of the pulses. If on palpation the pulse comes continually without interruption, this is a sign that the woman is pregnant. This is a way of saying that the pulses beat strongly, and are like a full river flowing continuously.

Following this various ways of knowing whether the woman is carrying a boy or a girl, or twin boys or twin girls, or a boy and a girl, and so on, are listed. For example, if you want to know if it is a boy or a girl you set the woman to walk southwards and call to her. If she turns to you with her left side she is carrying a boy or with the right it is a girl. Another funny thing which is mentioned is that if during the pregnancy the woman's husband, who is presumed to be the father, grows an excrescence on his left breast the baby will be a boy, and on the right breast it will be a girl. I find this interesting because here something is happening to the man.

GUANZI CHAPTER 39

I would like to present a text now which is about the development of the fetus. It is very short, and in a chapter in the Guanzi which has nothing to do with physiology or medicine. Guanzi chapter 39 is an interesting chapter about many things, but all of which have something to do with cosmic identity and with what happens on earth and inside the human body. There is a full passage on the coming of life, on what gives life and makes it grow. This is not from a medical or anatomical point of view, it is from a more ethical or cosmological point of view. These things were definitely associated in early Chinese thought.

> 'A human being is water. When essence (*jing* 精) and *qi* (氣) of male and female unite, water flows between them and assumes a form. At the third month the resulting fetus begins to suck. What does it suck? The answer is the five tastes (*wu wei* 五味). What do these five tastes produce? The answer is the five *zang* (*wu zang* 五藏). ... After the five *zang* have been formed, they produce the five constituents of the body (*wu nei* 五內). ... After the five constituents of the body have been formed, the nine orifices (*jiu qiao* 九竅) are developed. ... By the fifth month the fetus is fully formed; in the tenth month it is born.' (Guanzi chapter 39 based on Rickett's translation)

When it says a human being is water it does not mean the water element. There is a lot of blood inside the human body which flows and makes life in the likeness of the water which flows inside the earth, so perhaps that is a possible interpretation. However, in the next sentence water is also seen to represent a sexual background. Water is the rain which comes from heaven and the clouds, and the interplay of clouds and rain is seen as sexual intercourse. If you know the Mawangdui funeral banner, in the central disc of the lower part where the two dragons, *yin* and *yang*, are crossing, you find water flowing down and starting the process of producing the ten thousand living beings.

The second sentence says: 'When essence (*jing* 精) and *qi* (氣) of male and female unite, water flows between them and assumes a form'. This is an idea which was current at this time around the 2nd century BCE, that water is a kind of intermediary between what has form and what does not. Water is able to take all forms but has no form itself. There is water coming from the merging of essences and *qi* of male and female, so the river becomes living water, takes form and becomes the beginning of life.

After this the text abruptly says: 'At the third month the resulting fetus begins to suck.' We have to understand that the baby has not begun to be suckled by the mother, but that the fetus of three months now has the ability to take in nourishment. This nourishment is from the five tastes which then produce the *zang*. This is a very general process, but after that an association is made which is not found in medical texts. It says the sour produces the spleen, the salty produces the lung, the acrid produces the kidneys, the bitter produces the liver and the sweet produces the heart. This is completely different from what we are used to. However, the important thing here is to understand that all this process begins from the third month, with three being both the actual time of three months when the embryo becomes a fetus and a symbolic number. Symbolically three is a transitional number, in order to pass from one thing to another we need to pass through three. For instance, I need three years to complete the mourning for a parent. When a new baby was born in ancient China they were not sure that it would survive, so they waited three days before they cared for it. Three days can possibly be understood as twenty-six hours: a full day and one hour representing each of the other days.

In this text the third month of gestation is both real and symbolic. Something happens from the moment the water, made from the essences and *qi* of the parents, begins to take on a form. The fetus is able to start nourishing itself by the five tastes, and what it builds are the five *zang*.

'After the five *zang* have been formed, they produce the five inner constituents of the body (*wu nei* 無 內).'

These are the various parts of the body, such as bone, flesh and skin, related to each of the five *zang*. These five 'constituents' are presented in a completely different way and with different names and associations from the *zang* as they usually appear in medical texts. The spleen produces the diaphragm, the lung produces the bones, the kidneys produce the brain, the liver produces the skin and the heart produces the flesh. But what is important is that the relationships are alike. Each of the five tastes and five specific qualities of the essences allow the development of one of the five *zang*. And each of the five *zang* allows the development of one of the five constituents of the body. Then the process continues with the opening towards the outside:

'After the five constituents of the body have been formed, the nine orifices (*jiu qiao* 九 竅) are developed.'

This is the idea of making something appear, or come forth, and there are more strange associations here linking the spleen with the nose (the nose being the centre of the face), the liver with the eyes, and the kidneys with the ears. After this the text becomes very unreliable and there are some versions which relate the lung to the mouth and the heart to the lower orifices, while another version links the lung to the lower orifices and has nothing for the heart.

'By the fifth month the fetus is fully formed; in the tenth month it is born.'

Here the 'fifth month' is often amended to the seventh month. Also, there is no actual character for 'fetus', the text just says 'at the fifth' or whatever month it is.

From this text we see that the 'building' starts with

the most internal composition, the water, the ability to take a form, the five *zang* and the five constituent parts of the body, and then moves from the depths outwards to the surface and the nine orifices. This is the same movement as we will see in Lingshu chapter 10. But before that I just want to quote you the end passage of the text:

'The eyes see, the ears hear and the heart is able to reflect. What the eyes see is not limited to the sight of mountains and peaks. They may also examine what is indistinct and minute. What the ears hear is not limited to the sound of thunder and drums, they may also examine the sound of a baby's cry. What the heart reflects about is not limited to understanding what is coarse and gross, it may also examine what is fine and subtle (literally the secret marvel).' (Translation based on Ricketts)

The sense organs, which are the most complete achievement of the body, are able to perceive not only big and obvious things but also that which is not seen or heard directly. The production of a human being implies a destiny not just to comprehend the obvious, but to use the fullness of blood and *qi*, spirits and all the sensory faculties to go further than what is easily perceptible. The heart or mind can be used to think about what is really important in life and what is the subtle mystery of life.

Question: Do the Chinese differentiate between using the word fetus or baby?

We will look at this later because several characters are used and sometimes they are used with a specific meaning, but the problem is that it is not consistent. There are at least three characters for embryo or fetus, and there are several expressions used for a newborn baby. Sometimes the character for fetus is used for what is related to the time after birth, but a distinction is definitely made between the baby inside the mother and the baby after its birth.

LINGSHU CHAPTER 10

Let us look now at the beginning of Lingshu chapter 10 where we find described the same movement which we have just seen in the Guanzi, starting in the interior and ending at the surface. What comes afterwards in the text of the Lingshu is a full presentation of the twelve meridians and fifteen *luo* (絡) along with all their pathology.

'When a human being begins life (*sheng* 生), first the essences are perfectly formed (*cheng* 成). When the essences are perfectly formed the brain and marrow are produced. The bones make the framework, the *mai* (脈) give nourishment. The musculature makes what is hard, the flesh makes the partitions. The layers of the skin are firm and the body and head hair grow in length.'

Cheng (成) is the idea of something being composed so perfectly that a form is taken and fully achieved. It means to be complete. Very often *cheng* is found in relationship with the character *sheng* (生) which means life, to give life, to make appear, to give birth and so on. *Sheng* can be the birth, but it might also be the beginning of life before any actual form is given, as for instance in the water image used in the Guanzi.

When *cheng* and *sheng* are used together in the same sentence, normally *sheng* indicates the impulse and initiation given for a new life, while *cheng* is on the side of the achievement of this process. *Sheng* is the start of a process which leads to *cheng*, the complete development of a life.

In Lingshu chapter 10 *sheng* is used to mean the beginning of life, the initiation of the process of creating a new living being. First a form must be taken and it is the essences which form something. This represents the achievement of something at this first level of essences. In this context it corresponds to the essences coming from the man and the woman which when they join together result in the perfect formation of something.

The whole of the text from Lingshu chapter 10 gives the same movement coming from the kidneys and the depths, with the brain, marrow and bones then developing, finishing with the skin on the surface. This is not embryology, it is just a symbolic description of the process of building the body from the innermost part to its full achievement on the outside with the skin and body hair. The text continues:

'As the grains enter the stomach, the ways of circulation (*mai dao* 脈 道) establish free communication, and blood and *qi* then circulate.'

When the grains enter the stomach perhaps this is finally a baby starting its own life, with its own stomach and process of self-nourishment, and its own circulation of blood and *qi*.

HUAINANZI CHAPTER 7

The following quotation is from the beginning of Huainanzi chapter 7, a text published around 130 BCE, which evokes the beginning of the cosmos:

'In ancient times when heaven and earth did not yet exist, there was only image without form. Dark; obscure; formless; soundless; unfathomable; profound. No one knows its gate.'

From this inchoate state we have the beginning of the world of heaven and earth and the appearance of all living beings. But the point of chapter 7 is to examine the vital spirits of a human being: what makes a human being human, and what makes him or her at one with the cosmos, beyond life and death. Heaven is father and earth is mother, *yin yang* is the principle, and the four seasons are the regulator. Following from this the text describes the conception of a human being in the likeness of the cosmic process. It starts with the text which is found at the beginning of Laozi chapter 42 and continues with a short presentation of each of the ten months of gestation:

'One gives rise to two, two gives rise to three, three gives rise to the ten thousand beings. The ten thousand beings lean on the *yin* and embrace the *yang* and the powerful blending of *qi* makes harmony.

Therefore it is said:

At one month it is a rich paste (*gao* 膏)

At two months it is a bulge (*die* 胅)

At three months it is a fetus (*tai* 胎)

At four months it has flesh (*ji* 肌)

At five months it has sinews (*jin* 筋)

At six months it has bones (*gu* 骨)

At seven months it is complete (*cheng* 成)

At eight months it moves (*dong* 動)

At nine months it quickens (*zao* 躁)

And at ten months it is born (*sheng* 生)

As the bodily form becomes complete

(*xing ti yi cheng* 形體以成)

The five organs take form

(*wu zang nai xing* 五藏乃形)

Therefore, the lung masters the eyes

The kidneys master the nose
The gallbladder masters the mouth
The liver masters the ear
Those on the outside are for the external expression
Those on the inside are for the inner organisation
Opening and closing, expanding and contracting
Each has its regulation and rules.'

I insist upon the 'therefore' in the translation because we have to understand that in the vision of the Huainanzi there is a link between cosmic and human generation. If the beginning of cosmic life is really like this then the beginning of human life has to be similar. This is the reason why there are ten months, with the number ten reminding us that a woman will give birth at the end of ten lunar months. Ten fits with human nature because in the perspective of the Huainanzi, and many other texts from the 2nd century BCE, the vision of the universe was such that everything was in resonance and related to everything else. This is the period of time when the system of correspondences was established along with the final organization of the cosmology of the *wu xing* (五 行), the five phases or elements. If reality is truly like that, then everybody and every phenomenon is linked in a network of complete correlation with every other thing. The correlations are infinite. So not only do we have all these associations and relationships but we also have the complete pattern for the development of life through *yin yang* and the five elements. What occurs at the cosmic level also occurs on all other levels. It is not exactly an image of microcosm and macrocosm, but it is something similar with the same processes happening at each level.

Any manifestation of life, any event or circumstance, is the expression of a specific activity of *qi*. From that a lot of other things ensue. The Huainanzi says that if we observe the duration of the gestation period in mammals carefully we can learn something about their true nature. It is not by chance that a female human being gives birth after ten natural revolutions of the moon. It is not by chance that a female tiger gives birth after seven months. Numbers are not an abstraction, they are a reality of time and a quality of *qi* which give an indication of the characteristic qualities of each species. So for many reasons ten is the number for human beings.

The Huainanzi was composed in the second half of the 2nd century BCE and at that time a human being was perceived as the ultimate creation of heaven and earth, the most achieved of all the productions of nature. Ten is a number which expresses this perfection because all the stages of the development of life from one to nine have been completely fulfilled. In ten, all those transformations are gathered into an ideal unity. Ten is the number of everything which is perfectly differentiated and well organized, but which is also a unity. The character for ten (*shi* 十) is also composed in a very satisfactory way from this point of view. There is one vertical and one horizontal stroke, joined together by a crossing. In some circumstances *shi* can be used to mean perfect or complete. Ten months fit very well with this image of the perfect development of life, and a human being as the most achieved creation of life.

In Suwen chapter 1 the natural duration for a man's life is given as one hundred years, which is ten times ten. This is actually stated in other books including the Book of Rites. Ten is the basic number to represent a human being and the total number of the souls in a human being is ten: seven *po* (魄) and three *hun* (魂). These numbers were given to the *hun* and *po* at this time. Before the 2nd century BCE *hun* and *po* did exist but no specific numbers were attached to them.

For all these reasons a new human being needs ten months gestation. Ten is the number for a human being and ten is the number for the complete perfection of the achievement of life. The Book of Rites tells you what you are supposed to be and do at ten years old, twenty years old and so on. For instance, at seventy years, which is ten minus three, you start to prepare for death. This means retiring from public life, preparing your coffin and so on.

Let us look a little more closely at the first three months as described in the Huainanzi chapter 7 because the characters are really interesting.

'At one month it is a rich paste (*gao* 膏)
At two months it is a bulge (*die* 胅)
At three months it is a fetus (*tai* 胎).'

In the first month we have *gao* (膏). We know this character from Bladder 43, *gao huang shu* (膏 肓 輸). It is made up of two parts. The lower part is the flesh radical (月) indicating that it is something happening in a body made with flesh and blood. The other part is the phonetic (高) which has the meaning of something which is high or elevated. *Gao* is used for something having the consistency of a paste. In modern Chinese it is used for toothpaste for example. When we look at classical medical books we find *gao* used in several different ways, but an important one is as a heavy liquid or paste which is very rich in essences, something between a fluid and a paste. If you look at Lingshu chapter 36 or similar texts you find it linked with body fluids, but with the heaviest and richest part of them. It is something which is able to enrich the brain and marrow and even the sperm. We can call it a 'constitutive grease' or a 'fertile paste'. The understanding at that time was that this substance reached everywhere inside the membranes and tissues, and was a condensation of essences.

What exists in the first month therefore, is something still liquid but which nearly has a form, although not yet. It is no longer a flowing liquid because it is in the process of condensing into a paste. This paste is specifically rich in life-giving essences and endows the substance with the ability to be transformed. I have translated it as 'rich paste' because 'paste' is not sufficient on its own, and 'rich' gives a good indication of the richness and fertility of the essences, and the potential for life that is inherent in the character.

The character which is used for the second month is a very rare one, *die* (胅). You do not find it in normal dictionaries. It is made with the flesh radical again (月), and the phonetic part on the right has the meaning of to lose. The meaning of *die* is something which protrudes, a bulge. First there was a formless paste, but now there is a surge, a bulge. In comparison with the paste it is as if there was a yeast in the paste making it rise or expand into a bulge. So the meaning of *die* is that there is not only the paste but the paste plus a kind of inflation. But there is not yet the form of a fetus.

In the third month there is a fetus, *tai* (胎). The character for fetus is made with the flesh radical (月), and on the right-hand side there is the releasing or exhalation of *qi* (台). Below is a mouth (口), and above there is the emanating of *qi* (厶). Another character which has the same right-hand part, but with the radical for a woman (*nu* 女), is *shi* (始), the beginning of something. The beginning of life is well illustrated by the character showing the exhalation of *qi* and a woman.

The problem of translation is that *tai* (胎) is often translated by 'embryo' in daoist texts. For example, *tai* is used with reference to the 'embryonic respiration' (*tai xi* 胎 息), deep breathing and work on the *qi*, which is part of daoist practice. In medical texts *tai* (胎) mostly refers to the fetus which is formed in the third month, and other characters such as *pei* (胚) may be used for the embryo. Unfortunately in some texts, including some medical texts, *tai* is used as meaning embryo and *pei* as fetus. They are not concerned by the difference.

Nevertheless, we normally find a difference between what exists in the womb before and after the third month, and the most usual name for what exists after three months is *tai*, which corresponds to what we call fetus.

Something is different after the third month because there is the beginning of the specific building of the body of a new being which was impossible before. Other texts too have the first three months and afterwards another series. Now in the fourth month a precise structure starts to emerge. In the Huainanzi for the following three months (fourth, fifth and sixth) flesh (*ji* 肌), muscular forces, or muscular movement (*jin* 筋), and bones (*gu* 骨) are mentioned. After this in the seventh month something is achieved (*cheng* 成), since the bodily form is then more or less complete. What happens after this is more to do with movement. This process of putting into motion is also mentioned in some other texts. It is not that the fetus did not move before this time, but that now the movement is the main activity, and it moves more and more. In the eighth month it moves (*dong* 動), and in the ninth month it quickens and creates a kind of agitation (*zao* 躁). Finally, in the tenth month it comes out and is born (*sheng* 生).

Therefore in the description of these ten months there are several groups visible: the first three months for the beginning, followed by another three months for the bodily form, and then another three months for the movement and completion. Finally in the tenth month everything is finished. The passage ends with the following sentence:

'As the physical body becomes complete (*xing ti yi cheng* 形體以成), The five organs take form (*wu zang nai xing* 五藏乃形).'

Two characters, *xing* and *ti* are used together here for the body. *Xing* (形) is used for the body as the shape or form, and *ti* (體) is for the body as an organization of several elements or parts which make up a whole. So both characters may be translated by 'body', but not from the same point of view. *Xing* is a form, and *ti* is an organization. Therefore the text is emphasizing that all the bodily form with the organization of all its parts is complete at this time.

'The five organs take form' means that they are functioning normally and fully. The form reveals the activity of the *qi*. If the form is perfect, the activities of the *qi* are perfect. In Lingshu chapter 47 this idea is considered by looking at the form of each organ. For instance, if the heart is too large or too small or a little too high up in the chest, there will be a tendency to this or that disease or disorder. The form of the organ and its position reveal the good or bad functioning of the *qi*. The next sentences in the text are:

'Therefore, the lung masters the eyes
The kidneys master the nose
The gallbladder masters the mouth
The liver masters the ear

Those on the outside are for the external expression
Those on the inside are for the inner organisation
Opening and closing, expanding and contracting
Each has its regulation and rules.'

Repeated here are the relationships between the interior five *zang* and the exterior openings, with all the regulation of the exterior by the innermost forms. What we see on the exterior lets us know what is on the inside.

Huainanzi chapter 7 is interesting because it shows the same pattern as we find in other texts. Around the same time that the Huainanzi was written, at the beginning of the 2nd century BCE, various schools had ideas about the development of new life in the womb of a woman during the tenth months of gestation. It is not certain that they were medical schools as such, but they were schools interested in the enrichment and nourishment of life. In the Mawangdui texts found in the tomb near Changsha south of the Yangtze and dating from the middle of the 2nd century BCE, they found books of the Nourishing Life school including some medical books and some books on sexual arts and practices, and on the development of the embryo and fetus and the way to give birth. In these the development of the embryo and fetus was also made over ten months.

THE ZHUBING YUANHOU LUN 諸 病 源 候 論

We will now look again at the Zhubing Yuanhou Lun, a text which presents a month-by-month progress through pregnancy. We will also make a comparison with Sun Simiao and the Mawangdui manuscript which are essentially the same text with some variations.

FIRST MONTH

'The first month of pregnancy is called the beginning of the form (*shi xing* 始形). [The woman] must nourish herself with essences and cooked foods (*jing shu* 精熟), and choose sour tastes. It is therefore appropriate to eat barley (*da mai* 大麥), but she must not eat acrid and pungent (*xing xin* 腥辛) foods. This is called the gestation of the innate material (*cai zhen* 才貞). The *jue yin* of foot supports it (*yang* 養). The *jue yin* of foot is the liver circulation (*mai* 脈, the liver meridian) and the liver governs the blood. During the first month the blood flows with difficulty and no longer comes out, this is why the *jue yin* of the foot supports it. The point on the *jue yin* of the foot is found at the interval of the big toe, at the limit of the white flesh.'

The Zhubing Yuanhou Lun has a similar structure for each of the first three months, with a name given to the stage of development: 'The first month of pregnancy is called...', and so on. From the fourth month the formula changes a little and the 'is called' becomes 'begins to receive'.

In this text the character *shi* (始), which means a beginning, is used throughout. It is used from the first month up until the last month. For example in the fourth month the fetus is said to 'begin to receive (*shi shou* 始受) the essences of water.' When something starts it is always out of reach, and we cannot see or perceive the real beginning of anything. When the process of new life starts in a woman, nobody knows the moment, and perhaps nobody should ever know. What is important and what we are able to study are the beginnings of the evolution and the signs which we can read once things have already begun. This is exactly what is described here. We cannot say anything about the first beginning which exists in the mystery.

The text of the Mawangdui manuscript starts before the first movement by describing sexual intercourse in a very poetic way. It says:

> 'Therefore, to generate a human being, [a man] has to enter into the obscure darkness (*bei ming* 北 冥) and exit from the obscure darkness, and this begins the process of making a human.'

In other words, to generate a new human being there is a penetration which takes place in the obscure darkness and an exiting from that obscure darkness.

Of course this is a description of the movement of the penis in the vagina, but it is also described in such a way that the characters we translate as the 'obscure darkness' (*bei ming* 北 冥) are the same as are used at the beginning of Zhuangzi chapter 1 to describe the northern abyss in which the big fish Kun appears and then rises to become the phoenix bird, Peng:

'In the northern darkness (*bei ming* 北 冥) there is a fish whose name is Kun. Kun is so huge I do not know how many thousand *li* he measures. He changes and becomes a bird whose name is Peng.'

This is clearly a symbol of cosmic life, beginning in the depths of water and emerging into the light of heaven. It is an image of the beginning as an obscure darkness. It is both obscure and mysterious. The origin of life on earth is always in dampness, water, darkness and hidden in the depths.

In the Zhubing Yuanhou Lun in the first month there is just the beginning of a form (*shi xing* 始 形). We do not have to understand 'form' as a precise form, so it is not contradictory to the text of the Huainanzi chapter 7 which we saw previously. It is just another way of expressing things. In the Huainanzi there was a paste, *gao* (膏), which already had a form, but not a fixed or precise one. Here there is something which appears, but is a formless form, a substance, a material to be moulded.

Sun Simiao speaks of 'the beginning of the embryo' in

the first month (*shi pei* 始 胚). In another text he says:

> 'The child in gestation *(er zai tai* 兒 在 胎):
> In the first month, it is a embryo (*pei* 胚).'

The Mawangdui manuscript has an interesting variation. The first month is called 'flowing into the form', with the idea of something flowing into a mould. In ancient times there was almost no difference between a mould and the form it created. This is close to what we saw in Guanzi chapter 39 with the image of water flowing into something which makes it begin to take a form:

> 'A human being is water. When essence (*jing* 精) and *qi* (氣) of male and female unite, water flows between them and assumes a form.'

The image is of water flowing into a vase and taking the form of that vase, at least for a while, just as a human being is granted a body to live in for a while. Water is also the most common metaphor for *qi*. The concentration of *qi* is life and its dissemination is death. On earth life is first a condensation of essences which allows the *qi* to start working with them, shaping and developing them. The Zhubing Yuanhou Lun says:

> '[The woman] must nourish herself with essences and cooked foods (*jing shu* 精 熟), and choose sour tastes.'

The 'essences' here stand for the best quality food from which you can draw the finest essences in order to nourish the blood. A woman needs to keep a good balance between her blood and *qi* and we will see later on the pathology that arises when that balance is not kept. It is very important for the mother to have the best quality of essences for the renewal of her blood and bodily fluids, since they are part of the maintenance and nourishment of the uterus and of what it contains. A woman is not supposed to eat raw vegetables at the very beginning of a pregnancy. It is better to have cooked food because it is easier to digest and does not lead to stagnation of liquids and mucus, or cold. Nothing must disturb the blood and *qi*, and she must have the best quality of essences and blood, and also avoid becoming tired or doing anything that might block the relationship between *yin* and *yang* or blood and *qi*.

Some examples of appropriate food to eat at this time are given, for example barley. Then comes what is forbidden: 'she must not eat acrid and pungent foods'. Acrid and pungent are the taste and smell linked to the west and metal. A woman needs to eat sour food because the sour taste has the effect of gathering in order to strengthen the liver, especially in its ability to keep and store the blood. This is the basic function of the liver. At the beginning of gestation there is a need to increase the storing of blood, and to do that through the liver. By means of the sour taste the concentration and gathering of the essences is invigorated, but pungent and acrid have the opposite effect promoting diffusion and dissemination. So if the woman experiences pungent and acrid during the beginning of a pregnancy, then she takes a risk.

'This is called the gestation of the innate material (*cai zhen* 才 貞).'

Cai (才) is the natural quality of something. If you add the wood radical (木) it forms a character with the meaning of raw material (材). A raw material might be a piece of wood which you could use to make a table or something. But at the same time it is not so raw that you can do anything with it, since it has its own properties. If you make a container from wood, it is better not to put it on a fire because it will burn. A raw material does not have a precise form, but it has some specific qualities. If you remove the wood radical from the character *cai* it removes the material aspect, and you are left with the natural qualities or capacities. The various aptitudes and capacities are the raw material of a living being, their potential. When someone on earth starts the process of life there is already a natural endowment, an inherent nature decided by heaven. These innate qualities are not yet expressed, but they are nevertheless there. This fits with the theory of someone having an intrinsic, original nature. There is something already there, even if it is just the beginning of a form, even if it is just a kind of heavy liquid. There exists not only what is visible, but what is invisible inside, which is the natural endowment.

The character *zhen* (貞) is also very interesting. It is close to but still different from the character *zhen* (真) meaning authenticity. Authenticity is faithfulness to the origin. *Zhen* (貞) means something which is upright, and which is able to remain upright, and be constantly in the direction of what is right and pure, and the natural order of life. So with *cai zhen* there is the double idea of natural capacities and keeping of them in the correct orientation, of keeping the original purity of the potential to be developed. More than that, *zhen* (貞) has a specific use in the Book of Change. It is part of a group of four characters which are used for the four seasons. *Zhen* is used for the power of the winter. The virtue of the winter and the north is the withdrawal, or return to the most inner place in order to allow transmutations and transformations internally and to prepare for the renewal. In the Book of Change it often indicates the moment when a new situation is in gestation. It is a time to consult the oracle and take the correct orientation. The basic idea of this expression is that we already have something which is given which is pure and right and upright, because it is natural. It is up to us to maintain that in the correct way. In gestation it is up to the mother to adopt the best behaviour for maintaining the correct development of the child.

In his text Sun Simiao changed the character *zhen* (貞) for *zheng* (正), to be correct or to rectify. This is the same idea, that all the innate qualities and the natural endowment are kept correctly and uprightly. When a new life starts it is not only a matter of the father and mother, there is also something else which is a presence and an instigation, the possibility of starting a process of life which is given by heaven, or nature, or the natural order (*tian* 天).

Question: Is this zhen (貞) *connected with the will of the kidneys?*

It is not used in the Book of Change like that. What we have is a *yin* movement of condensation, which is the initial movement. First there is the concentration of essences, the coagulation of blood through the kidneys and the liver, which is the movement to be protected. It is related to the liver and the liver meridian because it is a question of blood. The liver is really the first to change, so the risk is also there. If it heats the blood too much for example, that is a risk. This is why it is so important to check the food which makes the *qi* of the five *zang*.

'The *jue yin* of the foot supports it (*yang* 養). The *jue yin* of the foot is the *mai* of the liver, the liver governs the blood. During the first month the blood flows with difficulty and no longer comes out, this is why the *jue yin* of the foot supports it. The point on the *jue yin* of the foot is found at the interval of the big toe, at the limit of the white flesh.'

The location of a point is given for each of the meridians

cited during the first nine months of pregnancy. I do not think these are points which have to be needled during pregnancy, because that would be a contradiction to what is said in a lot of other texts. Personally I feel they are points given to identify the meridian for sure. What we find in a lot of books, Sun Simiao for instance, is that because we have to be very careful with the liver and the liver meridian at the beginning of gestation, we are not supposed to needle or apply moxibustion on it during the first month. Sun Simiao adds:

'The *jue yin* of the foot internally is related to the liver and the liver masters the muscular movement and the blood.'

He says that in the first month the blood flows with difficulties, so the woman is not supposed to move with a lot of strength. If the woman makes a lot of muscular effort the blood will go to the muscles and less will be at the disposal of the uterus. But more important than the quantity of blood is the movement and activity of the liver. Muscular effort stimulates the liver and prevents it keeping the blood. As a result the blood cannot coagulate quietly inside the uterus. Sun Simiao even adds that it is better to sleep and rest and to be really calm and quiet. A woman should rest at this time, but later she has to move, as we will see later on.

Sun Simiao also adds that the woman must not have any fears. If there is a fear there will be disorder and agitation, and the fear will disrupt the essences and *qi*.

If there is no longer a connection between them there is a danger of losing blood or essences as there are not enough *qi* to manage and maintain the blood. The *qi* must be in good balance with the blood. Fear leads to a disruption of this balance, with the blood is no longer kept and transformed because the *qi* are missing.

This presentation of the beginning of gestation is similar in some ways to what is written at the end of Suwen chapter 8 after the presentation of the twelve officials about the formation of life:

'The supreme Way is in the imperceptible, change and transformation without end! Who then would know its origin? Alas, it disappears and one searches anxiously for it! Who then would know the essential? Oh, the anguish of actual situations! Who then will know how to act properly?

'Countless appearances and disappearances, out of which come forth the finest threads, fine threads that multiply until you can weigh and measure them. By the thousand and ten thousand they increase and grow, through development and growth creating the bodily form, governed by rules.'

(cf: The Secret Treatise of the Spiritual Orchid, Monkey Press, 2003)

First there is the mystery, and at the beginning of life there is something which is finer than the finest silk thread. But there is accumulation, and through the form taken by accumulation there are rules which were already there, so a form and organism are given, as was said in the Huainanzi, the body with its organization, *xing ti* (形體). This is not only the form, but all the organs with the five *zang* as the organizing principles.

SECOND MONTH

For the second month of pregnancy the same descriptive expression is used in the Mawangdui manuscript, the Zhubing Yuanhou Lun and Sun Simiao, it is the beginning of the rich paste, *shi gao* (始膏). We saw *gao* (膏) used in the first month of the Huainanzi chapter 7, but in these three specifically medical texts it is used for the second month. The expression is not so anatomically precise that this is a contradiction. The first month is the beginning of taking a form, and by the condensation and the concentration there is the constitution of this fertile paste which is full of essences and life, and full of the possibility of making an embryo. So it is not very different. The Huainanzi is more poetic with the image of the paste and the fermentation inside the paste, but medical texts prefer a slightly different approach.

'The second month of pregnancy is called the beginning of the rich paste (*shi gao* 始膏). [The woman] must not eat acrid and pungent (*xing xin* 腥辛) foods. She must stay quiet and avoid sexual relations, because that could cause pains in the one hundred joints. It is also called the beginning of storing or treasuring (*shi cang* 始藏). The *shao yang* of the foot supports it. The *shao yang* of the foot is the circulation (*mai* 脈) of the gallbladder and it is governed by the essences (*zhu yu jing* 主於精). In the second month, the essences of the child are perfectly formed (*cheng* 成) in the uterus and this is why the *shao yang* of the foot supports it. The point of the *shao yang* of the foot is located behind the root articulation (metatarso-phalangeal joint) of the little toe, one *cun* above the supporting bone (*fu gu* 附骨), right in the hollow.'

This is the same pattern of description as for the first month. As far as the food and tastes are concerned the woman is supposed to help the continuation of the concentration of essences and blood, and avoid anything which may disturb this movement and stimulate the *yang* movement of expansion and spreading outside too much. You will notice a little difference between the first and second months because in the first month the sour taste was recommended, but in the second month only forbidden tastes are mentioned. In the first month we were at the level of the *jue yin* of the foot, the liver meridian. The liver takes advantage of the sour taste for its own basic functioning and storing of the blood. Now in the second month there is no longer direct sustaining of the liver, but the woman must still take care not to disturb the gallbladder. It is not the *jue yin* of the foot which masters this period, but the *shao yang* of the foot.

We have to pay careful attention to these little details in the Chinese text. A repetition means something, and a change, however slight, means something, especially if it appears in all the various texts which we have. It will not be an error. I think the change here is because we are no longer in the *yin* but are now in the *yang*. We started with a *yin* meridian, but now we continue with the corresponding *yang* meridian.

Everything is done not to disturb the *shao yang* of the foot, the gallbladder. The gallbladder is one of the extraordinary *fu*, which is to say that the gallbladder has a special nature halfway between a *zang* and a *fu*. (cf: The Extraordinary Fu, Monkey Press, 2003.) It has the appearance of a *fu*, being a kind of empty pocket with a physical void inside and being physically full of something which is visible, the bile. But on the other hand it also deals with essences. It deals with liquids or fluids which have already been processed by the body and which are nearer to essences and to what is completely integrated into the body and used to promote the correct functioning of the whole physiology.

This is a big difference from the other *fu* of the digestive tract. For them there is a process of sorting which has to be made between what needs to be integrated and what has to be rejected. This is the reason why it is said in the text that the gallbladder is mastered by the essences or governs through the essences, *zhu yu jing* (主 於 精). *Zhu* is to master, *jing* are the essences and *yu* is through or by. It is through and by the essences that the gallbladder may act, and before there can be the beginning of a human form in the third month there have to be the essences capable of making such a human form. The choice and the gathering of the essences are what occurs in the second month.

All this is not to say that the gallbladder alone is responsible for the essences but just that there is a specific relationship between the essences and the gallbladder. On the other hand we also know that the natural movement of the *shao yang* gallbladder is one which starts with an impetuosity and has a spreading out movement. This is in the likeness of *yang* or male activity. A woman's sexuality is more concerned with receptivity, while a man is more of an activator. For this reason the gallbladder is easily linked with the movement of male sexuality, with the essences also being the sperm. There is a spreading out of the sperm, which is the same movement we can observe in the gallbladder or in the *shao yang*. This is another reason to make a link between the gallbladder and the essences. It is also perhaps the reason why some authors have said that in the second month the essences of the father, the sperm, are completely assimilated and integrated into the blood of the mother in the uterus, forming the basis for the essences of the child itself.

So, the second month of pregnancy is associated with the gallbladder and its meridian, the *shao yang* of the foot, and through them with the essences which constitute the embryo and start the new life as the rich paste which is the substantial form of the essences. Of course the Huainanzi does not state any relationships between organs or meridians and specific functions, but the process is not very different from the one developed in medical theory. In medical texts in the second month of pregnancy, the *shao yang* is acting in the woman like yeast working in the 'paste' and making it swell. The movement of life is there, the *qi* are working on the essences. The essences are represented, in the Zhubing Yuanhou lun, by the rich paste, *gao* (膏), which is full of life. Remember that in the Huainanzi chapter 7, the second month was characterised by a protuberance or bulge, like the swelling of a bread dough. But this movement in the essences may be dangerous if it is too strong and can break the concentration of the essences. Nothing must be done which may stimulate the impulse of the *shao yang* too strongly. The keeping of the blood, under the authority of the liver, must continue to be cultivated.

What a woman must avoid during the second month is every activity, food or emotional state which might lead the gallbladder or *shao yang* to become over excited and lose its ability to keep the essences. Because of this we understand that she must not eat acrid or pungent food because they are too dispersing, and that she must stay quiet. In the Mawangdui manuscript it says 'the dwelling place must be still'. Certainly to remain quiet is to remain in quiet surroundings, not only to sleep but to be at rest generally, without distraction or excitement. This is the reason why sexual intercourse is discouraged. We may read this as meaning forbidden, or to use techniques which minimize the excitement and calm the spirits during intercourse. The point is just to avoid tiredness and excitement because excitement will stimulate the vulnerable *shao yang* of the foot.

The situation in the woman's blood and *qi* at this time is that if the liver falls out of balance it become dangerous. The liver must be very quiet because the blood nourishing the liver is also the blood nourishing the uterus and embryo. When the *shao yang* is the dominant force the *yang* and activity are stimulated. Passions, desires and internal wind created by over-activity can arise. This internal wind and over-activity of the *shao yang* will lead to pain in the 'one hundred joints'. This phrase means all the body's articulations. This is the disease we know as migratory arthritis which is often linked to the *shao yang* meridian or the wood element.

In later texts and commentaries on this subject a link is sometimes made between the gallbladder and what is called ministerial fire. This is the fire of the triple heater and the heart protector. Ministerial fire is all the fire except that of the heart when it acts as centre of the person. The fire of *ming men* (命 門) is always called ministerial fire since although it is powerful and original it is not the leader of the personal life. The triple heater as ministerial fire is linked with *ming men* and linked with the distribution and quality of all the *qi* in the organism. The heart protector, as the minister fire, is the movement of the blood circulating everywhere to carry out the orders and influences coming from the centre of the heart, or the heart as a centre of the being.

Where is the gallbladder in all this? Being the *yang* side of the wood element the gallbladder is the beginning or *yang* aspect of spring, the moment of time which comes just after the *yin* of the winter, which is related to the kidneys. In later texts, the gallbladder was associated with the ministerial fire of *ming men* and was understood to be generated by it. The role of the gallbladder is therefore to express the fire of *ming men* by making it visible and pushing it into manifestation. At the same time it must sustain the fire of the heart, the sovereign fire, which is the son of the wood element of the gallbladder.

Here I disagree with Harper, even though it is a very good translation and an interesting work. (cf: Donald Harper, Early Chinese Medical Literature, the Mawangdui Medical Manuscripts, Kegan Paul International, London and New York, 1998) He says: 'For a boy there must be no exertion, lest the hundred joints all ail.' (Taichan shu, p. 379) I rather think that whatever the gender of the child, the woman who over-exerts the *shao yang* during the second month of pregnancy is at risk of developing pain in the joints.

Harper's interpretation may be that the pregnant woman already has an idea about the gender of her child, and must take care not to exert herself if she is expecting a boy.

'It is also called the beginning of treasuring (*shi cang* 始藏).'

This is the beginning of storing the essences carefully, deeply and actively, as if they are precious treasure. Inside the body what must be treasured are the essences since they are the basis and foundation of life.

'The essences are the foundation (*ben* 本) of a living body (*shen* 身).' Suwen chapter 4

The variation found in Sun Simiao explains why the essences which are just starting to make a new life, have to be treasured:

'The embryo begins to become knotted (*jie* 結).'

This is a kind of coagulation where the essences are bound together. The embryo forms a sort of dot. The image is really nice because in the first month there is something coming together, and in the second month there is a dot or a bulge. The something is no longer just a floating form, half liquid, half who knows what. There was a paste and then there is the solidification of the paste. The essences of the child are perfectly formed and cohere to form life. It is like when I eat, the essences which are in the food become my essences and are useful when they are integrated. They compose myself. Before that they are only the potential of life and its renewal.

We often find the image of the embrace of two essences to give life. Of course at first these are the essences of father and mother, as *qi* and blood if you like, or as sperm and blood. They have to come together to make one, and with that which comes from heaven they have the possibility of making new life. But the essences coming from the mother also have to be knotted together and concentrated enough to actually start the process of forming a new being. This takes place in the first and second months. By the second month the achievement of the first process and the composition of essences is accomplished, and the essences of a new life then exist.

Question: Are there texts which deal with preparation for pregnancy?

Yes. If you are well balanced and in good health, then the main instruction given is how to have sexual intercourse in order to create a boy or a girl. There are pages and pages on that! But generally speaking if the woman is healthy, she just has to keep healthy and well-balanced and avoid anything which unbalances the blood and *qi* of her liver, or weakens the kidneys or loses blood. If the woman has problems you have to work on those first. That is just logical. There is nothing which I know of that is written specifically on pre-pregnancy planning in the way you mean.

In several other texts advice is given as to what is appropriate for the second month of pregnancy. For example, the woman must calm her *qi* and maintain her spirits peacefully, stop desires, especially sexual desire, and not eat acrid food or ginger. Also, she should not eat any kind of food which is roasted or fried, because it might create heat in the blood.

Question: But ginger is used for pregnancy sickness.

Yes. But you know how some women just eat ginger all the time, which is stupid because it is too much and they create disorder in their system. Also, in the decoction for morning sickness you never have ginger alone, other ingredients are added according to the specific state of the individual woman. The diagnosis determines the formula.

So, the second month is the period when the *shao yang* of the foot is supposed to govern through the relationship of the gallbladder and the essences. It is also the period when the essences of the child are formed and become its own. We started with the liver, the *yin*, in the first month and we continued in the second with the gallbladder, the *yang*. We have the normal sequence of the beginning of life on earth: first the *yin*, then the *yang* based on that *yin*. First the essences, then the *qi* present inside them and working on them.

THIRD MONTH

The description of the third month in the Zhubing Yuanhou Lun is much longer, in fact by far the longest of all the months. During the third month we really have a potential child. I am not saying that it is now a person, because that is not the way the question is addressed here. We are looking at a text from more than fourteen centuries ago and from a completely different culture. If we want to solve our contemporary problems, for example in relation to abortion, we can find rich material for reflection in these texts, but not proof or resolution. However, in the third month, with the symbolic value of three, we now are definitely in the presence of a fetus which is the beginning of a distinct person, and that is why this fetus will be male or female and this is the starting point of his or her 'education'.

As soon as a fetus is composed with all the characteristics of a human being, the process of education starts. What passes to the fetus through the mother is now affecting a person and not just coagulating essences. The beginning of the person is the beginning of the heart/mind (*xin* 心), and the ability to receive influences at the mental level. So what the mother thinks and sees can influence the formation of the child's mind. This is the beginning of the 'education'. There were even treatises entitled 'Education of the Embryo' (technically the fetus) according to the usual translation. They existed as early as the Han dynasty (206 BCE - 220 CE). So, in this third month, the fetus is being formed and the mother starts to influence the heart/mind of the child.

'The third month of pregnancy is called the beginning of the fetus (*shi tai* 始 胎). At this time, the blood no longer flows, the image of the body (*xing xiang* 形 象) begins to develop through transformations (*shi hua* 始 化), but the determining principle (*yi* 儀) is not yet fixed. It changes according to the people [the mother] is exposed to. She must therefore seek out the presence (sight) of those who are noble and accomplished, eminent and royal, people who are beyond reproach and serious; but she must avoid dwarves, the deformed and midgets, all people of ugly and horrible appearance who look like monkeys. She must not eat ginger or hare (*jiang tu* 薑 兔) and she must not carry a knife or a rope.

If one wants a boy, one should practise archery on male birds, ride large horses (*fei ma* 肥 馬) in the countryside, go to see tigers and leopards and watch dogs running. If one wants a girl, one should wear hairpins and agate rings, and play with pearls and precious stones.

If one wants a child who will be beautiful and without reproach, look frequently at rings of white jade (*bai bi* 白 璧) and excellent jade, look at peacocks and eat carp. If one wants a child full of wisdom and strength, eat bull's heart and barley.'

First of all this stage is called 'the beginning of the fetus'. Exactly as is said in the Huainanzi chapter 7 in the third month we really have a fetus. What existed before was an embryonic or pre-fetal state, with not enough essences or clarified essences to make a form appear which will then become a child. Now menstruation has completely stopped and the embryo will take more and more of the mother's blood.

This form, or body (*xing* 形), is something which is always changing. A fixed form is a still life. The process of its formation has started in the third month because of the quality of the essences. The form is not yet totally taken, that will be done during the third month, so everything which can influence this process is important. Whatever the mother is exposed to is important because she will react if she sees an image of an ugly monkey man for example. What she has in her mind will influence the blood and *qi* working to make the shape of the embryo.

Xiang (象) is the image, or a pattern which is in action. It is not only the pattern but what you do with the pattern. For instance, if you have plasticene and a model, to mould something with the plasticene is *xiang*. *Xiang* is at the same time the model and the way that you make a form appear using the model. It is the pattern expressed in a living being. We can understand therefore why the image of the body 'begins to develop through transformations'. It is the realisation of the pattern through the plasticene, and this is made by the transformations and developments. The child in formation builds its body form according the human model, and also, in specific details, according to other models which are presented to it, beautiful or ugly, good or bad. These models enter through the mother, and through how her blood and *qi* are affected by what she sees, eats, thinks and worries about.

The idea of transformation appears here for the first time. S*hi hua* (始 化) means to begin to transform, or to begin to be transformed. This is the beginning of all the transformations which will lead to the complete achievement of the body, and after that will maintain the body and finally lead it to its end. That the character for transformation, *hua* (化), occurs here for the very first time is particularly interesting. No transformation appears in the first or second months, it only occurs here in the third month because the essences which enable the vital transformation of the embryo are now ready.

Through the potential and actual transformation there comes the making of a form, but it is not yet completely fixed and even the manner of the form is not completely determined. The character *yi* (儀) means a kind of pattern or model for a form, something like a template. The character *yi* also means a model or standard, a norm. The two *yi* (*er yi* 二 儀) are the two principles *yin* and *yang*, or the *yin* and *yang* lines of the hexagrams. With them you can model the possibilities of all couples. *Yi* is just the expression of this idea of a standard or model, implying that it might be *yin* and *yang*, male or female principle. In the fetus whether the child will be a boy or a girl is not yet decided.

'One must not eat ginger or hare (*jiang tu* 薑 兔)
and one must not carry a knife or a rope.'

One must not eat ginger because it is so powerful and
life-giving that to eat it could induce a proliferation or
superabundancy, resulting in extra fingers for instance.
The hare would lead to hare lips! There was a similar
idea in Europe. The literal and the symbolic go together.
The Chinese knew the state of the fetus because there
were many miscarriages and abortions, so there was
plenty to observe. The instruction not to carry a knife or
rope is linked with specific Chinese superstitions.

Because the sex of the baby is not yet fixed the
woman may act now in the third month to influence the
outcome. She could also have acted in the period before
conception. If a woman really wants a boy even before
she becomes pregnant she can start practising archery
on male birds.

'If one wants a boy, one should practise archery
on male birds, ride large horses (*fei ma* 肥 馬) in
the countryside, go to see tigers and leopards
and watch dogs running. If one wants a girl, one
should wear hairpins and agate rings, and play
with pearls and precious stones.'

Changing the blood and *qi* (*xue qi* 血 氣) balance, as
far as it is possible, is done through all that the woman
can see and experience. If a woman is in a mood to go
and see tigers or do archery, first there is an image in

her mind but there is also a feeling in her heart. The image, feeling and movement of her body will create the balance of her blood and *qi* and make it favourable to the creation of a boy. The balance of blood and *qi* is not the same for a boy as for a girl, so to influence this balance will affect the gender of the child. More blood and more *yin* will be the model for the body of a girl.

'If one wants a child who will be beautiful and without reproach, look frequently at rings of white jade (*bai bi* 白壁) and excellent jade, look at peacocks and eat carp.'

Jade is the prototype of all the virtues, in the sense that for the ancient Chinese essential moral virtues were found by analogy in jade. It is explained in the same chapter 39 of the Guanzi which we looked at earlier. White jade is the most pure, beautiful and precious of all jades. It is not only the jade it is everything which is evoked by the jade. In the form, colour and texture of the jade you find something which evokes and stimulates moral virtue in you. A peacock represents beauty among birds and a carp is a fish which is good and knows how to live a long time.

'If one wants a child full of wisdom and strength, eat bull's heart and barley.'

Question: Why are there references to barley and not to rice?

These are ancients texts and at that time rice was not so common in the north or in rural China. Rice extended through China over the centuries, but millet was the most widespread grain in ancient times. The God of Agriculture was Prince Millet.

The text continues:

'If the woman wants a child full of kindness and accomplished in virtue, she should regulate her heart and behave correctly. Be pure and empty (*qing xu* 清虛) in harmonious unity (*he yi* 和一). She should not sit askew on the mat nor stand leaning to one side, and when she walks she should not take roundabout paths (*xie jing* 邪徑). The eye should not look askew (*xie shi* 邪視), the ear should not hear depraved things (*xie ting* 邪聽), the mouth should not utter a bad word (*xie yan* 邪言), the heart should not have any bad thoughts (*xie nian* 邪念), she should not let herself be distracted by joy or anger, she should not let herself be taken over by worries and preoccupations (*si lü* 思慮), she should eat chopped up meat, she should not lie down askew (*xie wo* 邪臥) and she should not put her feet at an angle. She desires fruits and foods from the cucumber family, she is nourished by preserves of sour-tasting vegetables. She likes good odours (*fen fang* 芬芳) and dislikes bad ones. This is changing according to external images (*wai xiang er bian* 外 象 而 變).'

The cucumber family is comprised of things such as pumpkins and watermelons. Sour tasting vegetables are pickles and so forth.

Here in the third month of pregnancy, the education of the fetus starts. As soon as there is something which may be called the beginning of a fetus the process begins, and it is the mother who has to do the work. The education of the fetus means everything which happens to the mother, her behaviour, her way of moving, or putting her body at rest, singing, having emotions, or any kind of idea in her mind or inner thoughts, all this will influence the fetus. It is specifically at this time in the third month that the model and form will be fixed.

Of course this process does not stop after the third month, but this is the peak time because after this something exists which can never change. Therefore the woman must regulate her heart and behave correctly. If she is out of kilter in any way it is a sign of the state of her mind as well as her body, and the circulation of her *qi* will not be totally upright. This is very important for the model of blood and *qi* which is forming the child during this period. To be in harmonious unity, *he yi* (和 一), is to be in a state of concentration without stress and without over thinking. It is not a time to be disturbed by anything because somewhere or somehow this will affect the baby. This was known before psychoanalysis!

The same character which is used for perverse or evil *qi, xie* (邪), is used in all these contexts to mean askew, depraved, bad, or perverse. It is the contrary of upright and correct, *zheng* (正). Everything which is not upright is deviated.

'This is changing according to external images (*wai xiang er bian* 外 象 而 變).'

This is a way of saying that all the changes which occur during the formation of the child are made according to everything which the woman is exposed to. We can also say that it is changes resulting from inner images and how all these images are experienced inside.

'The heart master (*xin zhu* 心 主, *jue yin* of the hand) supports it. The heart master is the vital spirits (*jing shen* 精 神) present in the vital circulation (*mai zhong* 脈 中). Internally it is dependent on the heart and can mingle indistinctly with the spirits (*hun shen* 混 神). This is why the heart master maintains it. The point of the heart master is located on the horizontal line behind the palm.'

We know that the heart master is responsible for the circulation of the blood, the *xue mai* (血 脈). We also know that it is through the blood and its circulation that the spirits of the heart are present everywhere in the body. The blood is not only the nourishing fluid but what carries the power and presence of the spirits. The heart master masters the blood circulation, so it is indistinguishable from the spirits because the spirits are present through the blood. When we are moved by an emotion in the centre of our hearts then the blood changes. Therefore anything passing through the blood, the quality of the essences and food as well as the emotions and the quality of the vital spirits and the tranquillity and peacefulness of the heart, will be very important in the construction of the fetus. Sun Simiao adds to these observations that the woman has to pay attention not to feel any sadness or affliction, not to have any worries or concerns, to have nothing to make her afraid or to agitate her.

It is worth noting that there are no forbidden tastes here in the third month, just tastes the woman may desire. Concerning the question of special cravings in the pregnant woman, some texts and later commentators say that a woman's cravings reveal an emptiness in one of the *zang*.

The last paragraph on the third month is about the pulses:

'When one takes the pulse of the pregnant woman, if one finds it slippery and lively (*hua ji* 滑疾) and on strong pressure under the finger it disperses (*san* 散), then the child is already three months old.'

It is true that those who try and determine the sex of a baby by pulse palpation usually say the easiest period to do that is the third and fourth months. In the sixth month is it more difficult to tell from the pulses than earlier on in the pregnancy.

In the third month of her pregnancy the woman must have enough blood to nourish the fetus as it takes form and undergoes the transformations. She also has to keep the balance of essences and blood in all the organs in her body, and avoid any kind of agitation. Some commentators would say that it is because the heart protector is involved here with ministerial fire that the woman must avoid agitation due to passions, desires and so on.

In other texts sexual relations are also discouraged during the third month. Some say this is because the differentiation between male and female is not yet made, and also because sexual relationships will create agitation in the ministerial fire and heart protector which should remain calm and quiet, so that everything which touches the fetus will be clear and upright.

Some texts also state that if a woman does not behave correctly and follow all the recommendations, she will be increasingly imbalanced and prone to difficulties, and her delivery may be difficult. We know that at that time a difficult delivery often meant death. Agitation in the third month, through desire or emotion, or sexual excitement, would cause the essences to deteriorate. The fire burning the essences would lead to a stasis or blockage of the blood with the *qi*, and that might have resulted in a situation or a difficulty when the baby was born.

Morning sickness at this time is caused because the fetus is taking the mother's essences and blood. A counter current is created by the fact that the blood is below but there is an imbalance between the blood and the *qi*, especially at the level of the liver and stomach, or the *chong mai*, depending on whether you want to talk of organs or meridians. There is a pressing up onto the stomach leading to morning sickness. During this time it is therefore highly recommended that the woman avoid anything which might harm the stomach, and to pay a lot of attention to food or coldness or whatever generates phlegm or stagnation of liquids.

Question: Is there any link with or mention of Kidney 9, since we use this point at the end of the first trimester because we think it gives the fetus more blood.

That is not found in this kind of text. But of course you can use this point if it is necessary. Its relationship with the *yin*, the blood, is well known by the fact that it is the *yin wei mai* point.

FOURTH MONTH

In the fourth month we start from a new level because after the third month there is a real fetus. A human shape is established containing the potential of the vital spirits, and the beginning of a little human being, boy or girl. At this time all the essences are well composed and are able to make a living being appear, so there is a continuation of the development of the meridians, and the appearance of the succession of the five elements. First is water followed by the natural sequence of the elements. We will see later that this has nothing to do with the order of the succession of the meridians. The correspondence between the months of the pregnancy from the fourth to the ninth and the elements is an ancient one because it appears in the Mawangdui manuscript. It is at least as old as the beginning of the 2nd century BCE.

'In the fourth month of pregnancy, [the fetus] begins to receive (shi shou 始 受) the essences of water (shui jing 水 精) to form (cheng 成) the blood circulation (xue mai 血 脈). It is appropriate [for the woman] to eat rice (non-glutinous rice, dao jing 稻 粳) and to drink fish and wild goose broth (yu yan 魚 雁). This is called making the prosperity blossom (sheng rong 盛 榮) to make the ear and eye communicate (tong 通) and to make the meridians and connections (jing luo 經 絡) circulate (xing 行). When she washes, she must avoid cold and heat. The shao yang of the hand supports it.

The shao yang of the hand is the circulation of the triple heater, which depends internally on the fu (附). In the fourth month the child's six fu continue their formation (shun cheng 順 成) and this is why the shao yang of the hand supports it. The point on the shao yang of the hand is located two cun behind the root articulation (metacarpo-phalangeal joint) of the little finger.

When one examines the woman who is four months pregnant and one wants to know if it will be a boy or a girl, if the left pulse is lively (*ji* 疾) it is a boy and if the right pulse is lively, it is a girl. If the pulses are lively on both the left and right, she will have twins.

At this time one must take good care not to disperse, otherwise the woman may risk problems after delivery. Why is this? Because the circulation (*mai* 脈) of the triple heater, *shao yang* of the hand, depends internally on the triple heater, so she must keep her body calm, harmonise the desires and tendencies of the heart (*he xin zhi* 和 心 志) and regulate the diet.'

This is the beginning of the cycle the five elements, starting here with water. The fetus is beginning to receive the essences of water in order to form blood circulation. So there is not only a succession of beginnings, but also an achievement. To say that blood circulation is formed here is not to say that it is then the same as in the body of an adult. It is to say there is something which is perfect, based on the model of blood circulation, but it will continue to develop. However, the basis is established.

In her body the mother continues the successive cycle of the meridians. In the fourth month, the *shao yang* of hand, the triple heater meridian, is specially important and active in the mother.

It is difficult to establish definite relationships between the succession of the elements in the fetus and the succession of the meridians in the mother. Most probably they are not linked and of two different origins. But there is a continuity from one month to the next, in that what appears and begins to settle and develop in one month will sustain what appears and develops during the next.

If the heart protector, responsible for blood circulation, was mastering activities during the third month, the time of the achievement of that work is made in the following fourth month. So in the fifth month we find the achievement of the *qi*, the *qi* being more related to the triple heater, according to Lingshu chapter 10. Progression is always made in several steps or stages. If the work of the heart protector is done in one month, it is during the next month that there is the achievement of that work. At the same time there will be another meridian and another quality of *qi* taking responsibility for another new beginning which is then achieved in the following month. This kind of chain effect is very characteristic of Chinese texts and is actually quite systematic. But nevertheless we must maintain the difference between the two cycles and between what happens in the body of the mother (meridians) and the fetus (elements).

'It is appropriate to eat rice (non-glutinous rice,

dao jing 稻 粳) and to drink fish and wild goose broth (*yu yan* 魚 雁).'

There are several varieties of rice but *dao jing* is non-glutinous rice. This and the fish and wild goose broth are foods which benefit blood and *qi*. Hence there is an overlap between the heart protector and the triple heater during the third, fourth and fifth months. Here all the blood and *qi* and all their circulations are completely reliant upon each other. In the fourth month the focus is on sustaining blood and *qi*. The circulation of the blood is made through the meridian, but there are also circulations between the organs and the orifices. It is better not to do anything which may hinder all these circulations from developing, and all the networks and relationships being put in place.

This period of a pregnancy is called 'making the prosperity blossom (*sheng rong* 盛 榮)'. Prosperity is a character close to *ying* (營), which means nutrition. Sun Simiao, instead of saying this, calls it 'making the prosperity of blood and *qi* (*sheng xue qi* 盛 血 氣)'. One way or another, to behave and eat correctly during the fourth month will benefit the blood, the nutrition, but also their blossoming and all their circulations.

The text continues: 'to make the ear and eye communicate (*tong* 通) and to make the meridians and connections (*jing luo* 經 絡) circulate (*xing* 行).' This is because to open the orifices there needs to be a relationship between the *zang* and its orifice, between the innermost and the surface. The *qi* need to carry all the nutrition and blood to the level of the orifices. To fully realise the network of the meridians all the quality of the blood and all the regulation of the *qi* have to come together to achieve the meridian and its *luo* (絡) connections. The model is the flowing of water at the surface and inside the earth. The water is the blood of the earth, and the flowing of the blood in a human body is modelled on water and is organized by the water element.

If we want to force a relation with the triple heater, it may be done through its mastership of the *qi*, and through the relationship between the *shao yang* of the hand and the heart master meridian because it commands the circulation of the blood. The blood circulation and the *qi* are just in an interior/exterior (*biao li* 表 裏) relationship which is the relationship we have between the triple heater and the heart master meridian, and which is perhaps the strongest of all the *biao li* meridian relationships.

The woman must avoid cold and heat in order to avoid any disturbance in her circulation and therefore in the making of the model of the circulation of the fetus. Cold will slow the circulation and heat will accelerate it, and both will give an incorrect pattern to the embryo. The fetus is building its own pattern through the mother, just as it built its own essences before even becoming a fetus. If the mother does not eat enough good food the essences of the embryo then fetus will be poor. If she does not regulate what she eats the model given to the fetus will be disturbed with the possibility of remaining disturbed for ever.

There is another aspect which is mentioned here, which is the formation of the six *fu*:

'The child's six *fu* continue their formation (*shun cheng* 順 成).'

Why do the *fu* appear here in the fourth month? Perhaps there is a symbolic reason because four is the appropriate number for forms taken on earth, and the *fu* deal with food coming from earth. The *fu* have a form, and they deal with concrete, solid forms. Another reason is that they are do to with passage, circulation and communication. They are seen as a set of communicating receptacles. It is important that everything passes through them correctly. Here the triple heater is seen as being responsible for the *qi* and for all movements ensuring communication and connection, and of course there is a very strong relationship between the *fu* and the triple heater. There may be something happening at the level of the orifices, but there is also this movement creating circulation through the *fu* which is another kind of connection. This is the reason why the six *fu* are here. One of the main functions of the six *fu* is to act as a communication channel and passage. At this stage they are on their way to becoming accomplished. They have something in common with the quality of *qi* which is at work in the fetus, which is do to with communication and the creation of the network of communication. We could also say that the triple heater encompasses all the *fu*. In the Nanjing the triple heater is said to have a special relation with the *yang qi* and thus the *fu*. This relationship is expressed through the *yuan* source points on the *yang* meridians which are related to the *qi* of the triple heater.

It is interesting that in several texts, including Suwen chapter 5, with any kind of communication the orifices are on one side and the *fu* on the other. There is a subtle communication through the orifices but there is a more substantial communication through the *fu*. There is a movement with the ascending of the clear *yang* and the descending of the unclear *yin*. Therefore we can understand that even if it is strange at first, there is a good reason to present the orifices of the ear and the eye, and the six *fu* at the same time. They are the ways of all communication at all levels, and have to be in the network of circulation.

There is a lot of advice given in other books about the woman remaining calm and not getting too overexcited, and about regulating and harmonizing the triple heater. She must eat enough, but not too much. She must stand up, but not for too long a time, be seated, but not for too long, or lie down, but not for too long. This advice starts in the first month. All these instructions are to improve the circulation of blood and *qi*.

In the Mawangdui manuscript, something rather specific is mentioned which is that she is supposed to eat rice and wheat, and mud eel, which is a kind of fish. The flesh and the blood of this fish are used to have an action on the blood. What is interesting is the last sentence in the Mawangdui text which says that eating these foods (rice, wheat and eel) refreshes the blood and gives clarity to the eyesight. But to whom? To the mother of course, but through the mother it builds the pattern for the child. This does not cool the blood but just keeps it fresh and circulating properly.

In the Zhubing Yuanhou Lun it is interesting that it is at this stage problems concerning delivery and afterwards start to be mentioned.

FIFTH MONTH

'In the fifth month of pregnancy [the fetus] begins to receive (*shi shou* 始受) the essences of fire (*huo jing* 火精) to form (*cheng* 成) the *qi*. [The woman] should rest and get up late, wash the clothes well, live in the most interior parts of the house, put on thick clothes, go out in the morning to breathe in the rays of heaven (the sun, *tian guang* 天光) to avoid the harmful cold. It is appropriate to eat rice and wheat and to make beef and lamb broths, which she mixes with Zanthoxylum ailanthoides (*zhu yu* 茱萸) and seasons with the five flavours (*wu wei* 五味). It is also called supporting the *qi* to stabilize the five *zang* (*ding wu zang* 定五藏). It is also said to be appropriate to eat fish and freshwater turtle (*yu bie* 魚鱉). It is the *tai yin* of the foot that supports it. The *tai yin* of the foot, the circulation (*mai* 脈) of the spleen, governs the four seasons (*si ji* 四 季). In the fifth month the four limbs of the child are completely formed (*cheng* 成) and this is why the *tai yin* of the foot supports it. The point on the *tai yin* of the foot is located three *cun* above the internal malleolus.

When one takes the pulse of the pregnant woman, if on strong palpation it is not dispersed (*san* 散), but is lively (*ji* 疾) without being slippery (*hua* 滑), she is in the fifth month. If the pulse is fast (*shuo* 數), she is heading for complications (deterioration, *huai* 壞). If the pulse is tight (*jin* 緊), there are severe abdominal pains (*bao zu* 胞 阻). If the pulse is slow (*chi* 遲), the abdomen is congested with dyspnoea (*fu man chuan* 腹 滿 喘). If the pulse is floating (*fu* 浮), the deterioration of the water produces oedema (*zhong* 腫).'

This passage contains a mixture of many things. There is the element fire, but what is meant by receiving the essences of the fire? We can understand it as meaning that in this new being, which is now on its way to becoming complete and taking its own real form, the five elements produce life one after the other following the *ke* (剋) cycle. The first element had to be water since everything starts when a form is taken on earth by water. Something is hidden in the depths of the damp ground when a small seed has to germinate in the darkness, and it is exactly the same in the womb of the mother. There in the darkness with all the damp and water something is hidden, but with a lot of nutriment surrounding it. So there is a necessity to start with water, and perhaps there is a necessity to continue with fire, to show the coming of life and something which originates in the darkness and mystery but which is destined to come out and appear.

Fire must also come next in the sequence because of the blood and the *qi*. As soon as the essences are sufficient to form something, a being appears and the first constituents of its life are blood and *qi* as representative of *yin* and *yang,* water and fire. If we want to try to establish some kind of relationship between the prevailing meridians in the mother and the acting elements in the child, we may say that the heart master meridian was prevalent in the third month and its work is accomplished by the blood circulation in the fourth month. The triple heater was prevalent in the fourth month and its work is accomplished by the *qi* here in the fifth. The *qi* are necessary for all movement which involves the four limbs, so the formation of the four limbs here in the fifth month is a preparation for all the movement to come. Muscular movement arrives in the sixth month. We can also understand that it is quite correct to find this formation of the four limbs in the central position since five is half of ten, and ten is the complete set of numbers. It is appropriate that the centre is at the natural number of the centre, five, and the centre obviously has a relationship with the spleen and responsibility for the four directions.

At this stage the woman has to protect her *qi*, and

sustain the complete formation of all the *qi* and their expression in the fetus. She must avoid external heat and cold by remaining inside and not exposing herself to extremes. This is not a confinement, and it is very nicely put in the text: to 'go out in the morning to breathe in the rays of heaven (the sun, *tian guang* 天 光)'. This conveys the idea that in the early morning when the sun comes out the woman may go outside if it is a sunny day and take advantage of the rising *yang*. But she must come back in before it gets too hot or before she catches a cold, and she must not go outside in the evening since the *qi* at that time would not sustain the development of the *qi* inside.

The Zhubing Yuanhou Lun also says the woman must 'wash the clothes well'. In other texts it says she washes herself well. The Mawangdui manuscript says she washes her hair. All of this is the idea of being clean and pure, with the notion of unclean and soiled things being no good for the *qi*. This is a period when the woman has to be very careful of the quality of the *qi* around her. This is not only for her own sake but as the builder of *qi* for the fetus. It is not surprising to find the seasoning with the five tastes among the foods recommended because we are in the realm of the spleen. The spleen must be nourished to maintain and stabilize the five *zang*. This has something to do with one of the main functions of the spleen, which is to distribute essences (the five tastes) to each of the five *zang* in order to sustain them.

The form of the five *zang* starts to be completely stable

and real in the fifth month, even if they will only be fully functional later on. There are several steps in their development, and at this time there is a differentiation of the five tastes in the fetus making this possible. Little by little the rest will be achieved. The main point here is the idea of the mother's spleen functioning perfectly in order to give the fetus the right pattern for its own process of distribution. It is the same *qi* which make possible the distribution of the essences to the five *zang* and the nutriments and liquids to the four directions.

As far as food is concerned Sun Simiao said that in this month the woman has to eat enough but not too much, and she must avoid too much dry food in order not to damage the centre, the spleen and stomach and the balance of damp and dry. Also she must not go out in the sun too much, perhaps to avoid overheating.

We can also see that the *qi* which are in the fetus are the *qi* coming from the five *zang* and called the five *qi*. The pulsating of the five *zang* in the fetus is also the pulsating of the organ responsible for the releasing of *qi* via the work of the essences in the organism of the child and future adult. By its nature the spleen nourishes the five *zang*, and the spleen (and stomach) provide them with their post heavenly *qi*, so that they are full, stable, and able to release their own *qi* and continue their own activities. The four limbs are also nourished by the spleen, because the spleen *qi* are predominant when the four limbs are formed in the fetus. One commentary on the texts from the Zhubing Yuanhou lun and Sun Simiao text says: 'The *qi* are able to transport and make movement (*yun dong* 運 動).' Transport is the same character *yun* (運) as the one which is usually used for one of the functions of the spleen.

As regards the foods recommended for eating, fish and freshwater turtle, I think this is because they are said to be good for nourishing *qi* and maintaining strength.

SIXTH MONTH

'In the sixth month of pregnancy [the fetus] begins to receive (*shi shou* 始 受) the essences of metal (*jin jing* 金 精) to form (*cheng* 成) the musculature (sinews, muscular movement *jin* 筋). [The woman] wants to be a little active, not remain completely quiet, to go out walking in the countryside, to go often to watch dogs and horses running. It is appropriate to eat the flesh of birds of prey (*zhi niao* 鷙 鳥) and wild animals. This is called metamorphosis of the lineaments, the spinal column and the muscles (*bian cou lü jin* 變 腠 膂 筋) to maintain the nails (*zhao* 爪), to strengthen the back and spinal column (*bei lü* 背 膂). The *yang ming* of the foot supports it. The *yang ming* of the foot is the circulation (*mai* 脈) of the stomach, it governs the mouth and eye. In the sixth month, the mouth and eye of the child are completely formed (*cheng* 成), this is why the *yang ming* of the foot supports it. The point on the *yang ming* of the foot is located two *cun* above *tai chong*

(太 衝, Liver 3).'

The metal element and its essences are linked here with the completion of the muscular forces and movement, *jin* (筋), while the *yang ming* of the foot, the stomach, is linked with the completion of the mouth and eyes. As we saw in looking at the fifth month, it is quite logical to have the development of the muscular movement as a consequence of the establishing of blood and *qi*. Everything must be done by the woman in her body and mind to support the best possible pattern for the development of the muscular strength and movement and the appearance, formation and completion of the four limbs in the fetus. She must move her body, and avoid remaining still for too long, but without exhausting herself:

'She wants to be a little active, not remain completely quiet.'

This was a very important instruction for women of rich families because they would generally stay inside and do little, but they needed to move around and go outside, even into the countryside. The woman must give the right pattern to the fetus and she also has to give this pattern through her heart and mind, and through her ideas and feelings. She therefore goes to watch horses and dogs exercising, because when you look at these animals running, you have a wonderful image of muscular strength and movement.

For the same reason, she must eat the flesh of birds of prey and wild animals because they have good strong sinews and muscles. A bird of prey even has a beak which is really strong and which is made by the same quality of *qi* as the muscular forces, and their claws are like nails, which are the outer manifestation of the muscular forces. As for wild animals, they know how to run and move and how to use their muscular forces. This is not called sustaining the muscular forces, but metamorphosis (*bian* 變), which is something more developed. *Bian* is change, but in the way of allowing the full development of something. Here the complete development of the lineaments, spinal column and the muscular forces is achieved through the process (*bian cou lü jin* 變 腠 膂 筋).

Cou is linked to the skin and the rhythm of the *yang qi* coming from inside and displayed on the surface. *Cou* is often seen in conjunction with the character *li* (理) in the expression *cou li* (腠 理), meaning the texture of the skin. The meaning of the character *cou* (腠) is a little bit difficult to explain because it is mainly found in medical texts. The right-hand part (*cou* 奏) conveys the meaning of to converge, to collect, to come together, in the likeness of tributaries converging toward a river. The left-hand part is the flesh radical (月). The character *cou* (腠) gives the feeling of the *qi* flowing and converging at the surface, in the skin. Thus, it may be related to the movement of the *yang qi* and the defensive *qi* which form the way in which the innermost displays itself on the exterior of the skin. For example, the lines on my hand are my destiny, and the way my skin closes its pores carefully is also part of a design and the expression of the correct movement of *qi*. This is the same thing as defensive *qi* or *yang qi* surging from the original *yang* and expanding outwards. The *qi* with the utmost *yang* quality are expressed in the body as the defensive *qi* (*wei qi*), as the great *yang qi* or *tai yang qi*, the first of the six levels found in the Shanghanlun, representing the defense, and the bladder and small intestine meridians. These meridians, most particulary the bladder, run on the back and the spine, in close association with the *du mai* and with the defense. We can also say that the strength of the defensive *qi* comes from the ability of the stomach, and the *yang ming* meridian, to digest well and provide the forces coming from the food.

In the context of the sixth month the idea is about the correct display of the *yang qi* which gives strength to the spinal column and to all the muscles attached to the spinal column for the development of all the movement of the four limbs. Therefore there is a complete picture of how to make the pattern of the muscular movement for the four limbs function well already formed in the fetus, and also the idea of nourishing and sustaining those muscular forces where there is a central attachment.

'To maintain the nails (*zhao* 爪)' means to maintain the external appearance of the same *qi* which enables the working of the muscular forces internally. In other words the same *qi* which nourish the muscular forces are responsible for the quality of the nails externally.

'To strengthen the back and spinal column (*bei lü* 背 膂).'

This passage of the text is nearly the same as in Sun Simiao:

'This is called metamorphosis of the lineaments (*bian cou li* 變 腠 理), to make supple and firm the muscular movement (*ren jin* 紉 筋), in order to nourish the strength (*li* 力) and to reinforce the back and spinal column (*bei lü* 背 膂).'

In the Mawangdui manuscript the text has been corrupted, but it must have been the same originally because some of the same characters are used.

In some later texts it is said that the woman must avoid an excess of sour in the tastes because an excess will restrain the development of the muscular forces by encouraging the liver in its function of storing. It is not appropriate to eat sour foods because they will stop the liver blood being delivered by the liver *qi* which frees the *yang* movement of the liver. But it is not forbidden to eat it, just in excessive amounts.

The relationship of the stomach meridian, the foot *yang ming*, with the mouth and the eyes is mentioned here in the sixth month. The foot *yang ming* meridian has a relationship with all the facial orifices since it starts at the eyes, runs along the nose, has a relationship with the mouth, and goes to the ears. I think the eyes and mouth are mentioned here to represent all the upper

orifices. The couple normally used for this is ears and
eyes, but for the stomach we must have the mouth.
Perhaps by citing the mouth and the eyes we have all
that is most subtle, the images and emotions passing
through the eyes, and all that is most substantial, the
food entering the body via the mouth. There is also the
opposition between the emission of everything which is
subtle and without form coming out from the eyes and
the reception into the interior of physical substances
via the mouth. The foot *yang ming* meridian is also able
to sustain the light of the vision which is alluded to in
the name of the first point of the stomach meridian,
cheng qi (承 泣).

The *yang ming* meridian obviously has a lot to do
with the mouth, and not just at the level of the mouth
itself but with everything which enters the mouth and
descends into the stomach. For the eyes the relationship
with the foot *yang ming* is local, but also comes from
the depths because it is connected to the quality of
the rich body fluids brought by the stomach meridian
which are important in the eye area. So one way or
another the *yang ming* is very present in the correct
functioning of the eyes and mouth. It is because the
yang ming is predominant at this time that we have
these two organs completely formed at the sixth month.
Or it could be that because these organs are formed
at the sixth month the *yang ming* is prevalent. It is a
process of observation and systematic development
according to a particular theory of medicine. Either way
it is important to maintain the correct functioning of

the foot *yang ming* and of the stomach for the mother. As Sun Simiao says, she has to regulate the five tastes, and eat sweet tastes without guzzling!

At this point in pregnancy many women do have a tendency to guzzle. If the mother eats too much she will damage her stomach *qi* and give a bad pattern to the fetus. All the circulation and operation of the *yang ming* through the orifices of the face will be damaged and may leave the woman open to difficulties in the delivery.

SEVENTH MONTH

'In the seventh month of pregnancy [the fetus] begins to receive (s*hi shou* 始 受) the essences of wood (*mu jing* 木 精) to form (*cheng* 成) the bones (*gu* 骨). [The woman] moves the body and limbs, without letting herself stay still, moving in extension and flexion, and she stays in a dry place (*zao* 燥). She avoids eating or drinking cold things. It is appropriate to eat rice (non-glutinous rice, *dao jing* 稻 粳) to tighten (*mi* 密) the lineaments (*cou li* 腠 理). This is called supporting the bones (*yang gu* 養 骨) and strengthening the teeth (*lao chi* 牢 齒). The *tai yin* of the hand supports it. The *tai yin* of the hand is the circulation (*mai* 脈) of the lung. It governs the skin and body hair (*pi mao* 皮 毛). In the seventh month, the skin and body hair of the child are already completely formed and this is why the *tai yin* of the hand supports it. The point on the *tai yin* of the hand is located behind the root articulation (metacarpo-phalangeal joint) of the thumb, at the edge of the white flesh, right in the hollow.'

This month has the double achievement of the bones being linked with the wood element, and the skin and body hair linked with the lung and lung meridian. It is very interesting and logical to find the bones following on from the muscular movement of the sixth month. We are not pursuing a systematic development from the inside to the outside. First there were blood and *qi* in the fourth and fifth months, then in the sixth and seventh months there are muscular forces and bones. The muscular movements come first because as we know even in Western medicine it is through muscular movement that bones become stronger. Bones get harder and harder because we move.

It is possible that the Chinese simply observed all this. There were a lot of miscarriages and many dead infants, so it was easy to see and they could also observe the process in animals. It also makes sense in relation to what is always said, that *qi* precedes form. Movement precedes form. First there is *qi*, the movement, and afterwards there is the form, which becomes more and more solid. It is very eloquent the way the text says 'moving in extension and flexion', because we have to move like this in order to support the completion of the bones. The mother moving in extension and flexion, activates her body and gives the pattern of movement in order to strengthen the bones in the fetus.

'She stays in a dry place (*zao* 燥).'

To stay in a dry place is to avoid dampness which may block the circulation of blood and *qi*. When we want to strengthen the bones, the muscles have to move, but the muscles also have to move because the blood and *qi* circulate well. It is something which Sun Simiao says: 'Moving in extension and flexion in order to transport blood and *qi* (*yun xue qi* 運 血 氣).'

The necessity of avoiding eating or drinking cold things is probably linked to the lung. To have too much cold in the stomach would damage the *qi* of the lung since the *qi* coming from the stomach and digestion rise to the chest and the lung, and therefore inhibit the strength and proper working of the hand *tai yin*. I interpret the relationship in this way rather than with the bones and muscular forces, although there is also some connection there. It is a lot more direct with the lung. Afterwards the text says that the appropriate food is rice in order to tighten the lineaments, so here we are definitely dealing with the skin and lung meridian. We are concerned with the *wei qi* (衛 氣), the defensive *yang qi*, which are so dependant on the good functioning of the lung for their ability to spread up to and through the skin and body hair level. The *yang qi* are under the mastership of the *tai yin* of the hand, the lung, so there is a complete expansion by the *yang* and *wei qi*, not only in the back and spine as seen in the sixth month, but here in the seventh month to the very outer limits of the body where the skin and body hair are. There is a logic in this. I am sure that the ancient Chinese knew the form of the fetus at each stage and that was certainly the basis of the construction of these texts, mixed together with a lot of theory and correspondences of course.

In the seventh month the woman must not only avoid cold food and drinks in order not to damage the lung *qi*, she also has to be careful with cold wind coming from outside, or any kind of danger from outside which might damage the lung *qi*. More than this, as Sun Simiao said, she has to avoid speaking too loudly because when one speaks one uses the *qi* of the lung. At the seventh month the woman has to preserve the *qi* of her lungs as best she can, not to speak loudly, and of course not to cry, shout or sob. She must also avoid being in contact with the cold. She must be careful to have good clothes in order not to let the cold enter and damage the *wei qi* and the lung. She is not supposed to wash her clothes for fear of catching a cold. It is always bad to catch cold, but here the consequences will be felt in the development of the fetus too.

The relationship between the teeth and the bones is the same as between the muscular forces and the nails, so here to support the bones is the same thing as to strengthen the teeth. It is the same movement.

'When one takes the pulse of a woman who is

seven months pregnant, if they are full (*shi* 實), big (*da* 大), firm (*lao* 牢) and powerful (*qiang* 強), it is a sign of life; but if they are deep (*chen* 沉) and fine (*xi* 細), it is a sign of death (of the fetus). In the seventh month, it can happen that the pregnant woman, for an unknown reason, has bleeding (from the upper orifices, from the nose, *nü* 衄) and turning muscles (*zhuan jin* 轉筋); these are called the bleedings (epistaxis) of pregnancy. If this is set off by sneezing it has nothing to do with pregnancy. The pregnant woman, in the seventh month can suddenly lose water in great quantities, this is because the fetus is about to fall (miscarry); this is because at the wrong moment the amniotic fluids descend prematurely on their own.'

'Turning muscles' are little muscular spasms. It is a pathology linked with the tendino-muscular circulations which are everywhere in the body. A description of these twelve circulations is found in Lingshu chapter 13. There is always the possibility of this twitching of the muscles along the pathways, but it is not felt everywhere at once.

If the bleeding from the nose is set off by sneezing then it has nothing to do with the pregnancy. But an imbalance of the liver with a counter current of *yang qi* can make blood come out at the upper orifices, usually at the nose, which of course is related to the lung. This disorder in the liver also makes a twitching in the muscles due to an insufficiency of blood. This kind of insufficiency and over activity of the *qi* can lead to what is in the uterus coming out which could mean the loss of amniotic fluid.

Question: Does the spleen play any part in this?

Sure, but it is because there is the pathology in the muscles and the bleeding is in the upper orifices and because it is a sudden loss of water that I myself would be more likely to relate it to an instability and imbalance of the blood and *qi* of the liver. If it was the spleen there would be no reason for it to be so sudden.

EIGHTH MONTH

'In the eighth month of pregnancy [the fetus] begins to receive (*shi shou* 始 受) the essences of earth (*tu jing* 土 精) to form (*cheng* 成) the layers of the skin (*fu ge* 膚 革). [The woman] harmonises her heart and breathes calmly (or keeps calm and at rest, *jing xi* (靜 息), without letting the *qi* go too far. This is called tightening the lineaments (*mi cou li* 密 腠 理) and making the complexion on the face shiny and smooth (*guang ze yan se* 光 澤 顏 色). The *yang ming* of the hand supports it. The *yang ming* of the hand is the circulation (*mai* 脈) of the large intestine, the large intestine governs the nine orifices. In the eighth month, the nine orifices of the infant are completely finished, this is why the *yang ming* of the hand supports it. The point on the *yang ming* of the hand is located behind the root articulation (metacarpo-phalangeal joint) of the thumb, right in the crease.'

Here the lineaments are the work of all the *yang qi* at the surface of the body. The layers of the skin are active in such a way that the pores may be closed at some times, and open at others. They act in such a way that the *qi* are able to retain all the liquids inside the body when they need to be retained, or to release them when they have to move outside. What is responsible for the way sweat comes out of the body or liquids are kept inside the body?. At the first level it is because the pores are open or closed. This happens because of the activity of the *qi* at the superficial level of the body. The *qi* acting at the surface keep the balance and ensure a good rhythm of opening and closing of the pores. They also keep the liquids in the right form and movement, working in such a way that if there is heat which needs expelling for example, it will be cleared out via the sweat. If there is no excess heat the *yang qi* will protect the body by keeping essences, fluids and *yin* inside.

With this process in mind we can see that there is not only the substance of the skin and the pores but also the presence of the *yang qi* which make up life at the surface layers of the skin. The *yang qi* make the skin supple and allow the pores to open and close. The correct movement of all the *qi* converging at the superficial level is seen in the texture of the skin and the lines of the hand, the *cou li* (腠 理). These things are just the visible depiction at the exterior of the movement of the *qi* acting at that level, but coming from the innermost self. This is one reason why the four limbs are very closely linked with the *wei qi* and the *yang qi*.

Cou li (腠 理) is difficult to translate. I have used 'lineaments' to keep the idea of lines, such as the lines we have on the skin, but it is not a good translation. The problem is that there are different translations according to the context because the expression is used with different levels of meaning. It can be used for the spreading of the *yang qi*, the *wei qi*, from the lower heater to the surface layers of the skin, where these *qi* are responsible for the good maintenance of the skin, the appearance of the lines at its surface, and also the appropriate opening and closing of the pores. We do not have an equivalent word in English or French for that. In modern Chinese *cou li* is usually used to mean pores, but without the idea of all the activity of the *qi* behind them, the pores alone are not the same thing. The pattern of our skin is really the rhythm of our life and what guides it.

One of the best texts which explains the meaning of *cou li* is at the end of chapter 1 of the Jingui yaolüe. This is a very important book of medicine, presenting a theory of syndromes and diseases classified by categories, with indications for treatment by herbs and remedies, and written by the same author as the Shanghanlun at the very beginning of the 3rd century CE. (cf: The Essential Woman: Female Health and Fertility in Chinese Classical

Texts, Monkey Press, 2007)

Li (理) means the veins seen in a piece of jade, of marble or of wood, which reveal the inner organisation and reality. So the character is used for the inner structure of something, for the natural order which presides over its constitution and evolution. An old expression, the 'veins of heaven' *tian li* (天 理) refers to the natural order in everything, to the principles giving it its reason to exist.

The essences of earth are linked with the completion of the layers of the skin and now in the eighth and ninth months there is the completion of the enveloping structure, the layers of skin and body hair. At this time the woman has to be careful to eat enough because she has to sustain the *yang qi* and all the body fluids and essences. She has to be tranquil and quiet, and breathe calmly because excitement and overheating would lead to sweat. When the text says: 'without letting the *qi* go too far' it is reminiscent of Suwen chapter 2 and the description of summer when one is supposed to let the *qi* go outside or escape in order to balance the heat:

> 'One does not let oneself be overcome by the sun, exerting the will, but without violence (*nu* 怒), assisting the brilliance of beauty and strength which thus fulfill their promise. One must assist the flow of *qi* which likes to go to the exterior (*wai* 外).'

This is for warm weather, but in the winter it is the opposite: 'One must avoid the cold and seek the heat, not letting anything escape through the layers of the skin for fear of using all the *qi*. Everything must be done according to the light of the sun.'

There is something similar here. A woman in the eighth month of pregnancy is quite tired, so she risks suffering a lack of blood because of what has been used to nourish the fetus. She is also at risk from a lack of *qi* because pregnancy is exhausting and she herself is so heavy. She has to take care of herself and act as if it were winter, saving her energy for the delivery. She needs to be calm and quiet and not move around too much. If she moves too much and runs about she will exhaust herself and sweat which would mean a loss of *qi*. Or the movement could be mental excitement or too vivid an imagination. The fact is that *qi* are lost from this and it gives a bad pattern for the construction of the layers of the skin in the fetus, because it is not only the building of the skin, it is the building of the process by which the skin will continue to be formed and maintained. It is the process by which the *yang qi* will act normally and regularly on the surface of the body by keeping inside what has to remain interior. The woman has to be very careful to transmit the right pattern to the fetus. Doing all that is called 'tightening the *cou li* (*mi cou li* 密 腠 理)'.

'Making the complexion on the face shiny and smooth (*guang ze yan se* 光 澤 顏 色).'

The special skin of the face not only has the strength

of the *yang qi* of defence, but also the full functioning of the *yang qi* because of its alliance with the body fluids. There is the *yang* activity of tightening, but with body fluids present which are able to give a nice complexion. This is interesting because I think the body fluids are quite important in the eighth month of pregnancy and perhaps they are one link between the *yang ming* of the hand and the nine orifices.

There are many relationships between the large intestine, the *yang ming* of the hand, and the body fluids. For instance, in Lingshu chapter 10 the *yang ming* of the hand is said to be responsible for the pathology of the body fluids and it is related to several upper orifices via its pathways. A good lubrication of the large intestine is needed for an easy transit of waste matter. The meridian, *yang ming* of the hand, and the *fu*, large intestine, are associated with dryness which, when in excess, damages the body fluids.

The nine orifices are described in Suwen chapter 5 as a passage for the *qi* in the form of water. Therefore, at the level of each orifice, the upper as well as the lower, there is not only all the communication of the *qi* but all the circulation of liquids and their eventual release. Fluids pass through the lower orifices, and through the upper ones, although usually nothing comes out from the ear. The upper orifices and the *yang ming* of the foot were connected in the seventh month, but here in the eighth month the nine orifices are linked with the *yang ming* of the hand because it is more related to the two lower orifices. It is directly connected with the anus anatomically and perhaps related with the bladder through its relationship with the lung and this deep relationship with the body fluids. The upper orifices are also related to the *yang ming* of the hand because of its specific pathways and qualities. It goes up to the face and several of its points help to open the orifices and stimulate the circulations towards them, assisting their good functioning.

All this means that in the eighth month the woman has to take care of all her body fluids circulating at the surface of the body through the layers of the skin, in the orifices and so on, because at this time the development of the pattern of the relationships between the *yang qi* and the fluids in the body is being formed.

Sun Simiao says the same thing: 'Avoid dry food but do not lack food'. In other texts it says the woman should avoid foods which are not very clean and also avoid dry and acrid (or pungent) tastes. Dry and acrid are the tastes related to the metal element. They are to be avoided because the woman must not damage the *ying* of the large intestine, and the liquids under their control. These tastes could diminish the blood of the large intestine or lead to diarrhoea. If the text was a systematic presentation of the correspondences with this section about the hand *yang ming*, the metal element and the acrid taste, we would normally avoid the bitter taste. But this is not the case here, so it is not a systematic theory which is being applied.

'When one takes the pulse of the woman who is

eight months pregnant, if they are full (*shi* 實), big (*da* 大), firm (*lao* 牢), powerful (*qiang* 強), wiry (*xian* 弦), tight (*jin* 緊), it is a sign of life; but if they are deep (*chen* 沉) and fine (*xi* 細), it is a sign of death.'

NINTH MONTH

'In the ninth month of pregnancy [the fetus] begins to receive (*shi shou* 始受) the essences of stone (*shi jing* 石精) to form (*cheng* 成) the skin and body hair (*pi mao* 皮毛), the six *fu* and the one hundred joints (*bai jie* 百節); all is complete. [The woman] drinks tasty drinks (*li* 醴) and eats sweet things (*gan* 甘). She loosens her belt and waits. This is called supporting the body hair and head hair (*mao fa* 毛髮) to increase talent and strength. The *shao yin* of the foot supports it. The *shao yin* of the foot is the circulation (*mai* 脈) of the kidneys, the kidneys govern continuity (*xu lü* 續縷). In the ninth month, the continuity of vital circulations (*mai* 脈) is completely finished and this is why the *shao yin* of the foot supports it. The point on the *shao yin* of the foot is located behind the internal malleolus, level with the arterial beating (*dong mai* 動脈) a little in front and below.'

'To receive the essences of stone' is an ancient expression because it exists in the Mawangdui manuscript. What is meant by stone here is a concentration of essences. If we take the *ren mai* points on the lower abdomen, from Ren 3 to Ren 7, their names allude to the origin and its manifestation as *yin* and *yang*. Ren 3 (*zhong ji* 中 極) alludes to the origin which exists behind the beginning, while Ren 4 (*guan yuan* 關 元) alludes to the *yin* and *yang* beginning together. After that there are two points, Ren 5 and Ren 6, which certainly allude to the richness and power of the *yin* and the *yang*. It is obvious that Ren 6, the sea of *qi* (*qi hai* 氣 海) in the lower abdomen, expresses the *yang*, so Ren 5 (*shi men* 石 門), stone gate, must express the *yin*. The character *shi* (石) means stone, rock, mineral, hard, petrified or barren. With another pronunciation, *dan*, the same character has the meaning of stone as a unit of Chinese measurement, a picul.

The image of a stone is used for infertility, a stone belly is a sterile woman. But it is also used in order to show the concentration of the essences and the taking of form inside the earth. Jade is understood as the essences of heaven concentrated in the bosom of the earth, and this is the reason why jade is considered the most precious substance and the pattern for all virtue. By analogy with that we can understand that a stone is a concentration of essences, and if it is well made it is full of possibilities and circulation and so on. It is a bit like the bones of the earth. We have bones in our body, and there are stones and rocks in the earth.

In the first month of pregnancy, the woman gathers the essences which are like a fluid paste or rich water.

In the fourth month, the child receives the essences of the water (element) to organize its blood circulation (*xue mai* 血 脈) on the pattern of the rivers and waterways on earth. In the ninth month, when the water element comes back in the cycle as stone, the vital circulation (*mai* 脈) forms a complete network present everywhere in the body and ensures the continuity between the origin and its manifestation in an actual life.

The fetus is no longer fluctuating without skin and definition, there is a completion with real limits at the enveloping layers of the skin and body hair, and these are signs that everything is finished. We understand this achievement in stone through these associations which come from the end of the 3rd century and the beginning of the 2nd century BCE, a period when the correspondences of the five elements were not yet well defined and the organizations by four, five and six were still mixed up.

Also, after the five elements we now have a sixth, or something which is not quite an element but almost. The problem is that when we speak of five elements or phases they have to be five in order to be what they are, which are the master categories of the cosmology. If they are not five they are no longer the master categories. But here in this context they needed a sixth element because they had another month to present. Here the choice of stone may be understood through the vision of stone or jade as a concentration and the taking of a definitive form, or as flowing water assumes a form in a receptacle or as ice.

This fits quite well with the idea of the completion

of the form by the definite border it has. At the ninth month, the completion is expressed by the external limit of the body at the skin. The skin, which is also the place where all the exchanges between outside and inside take place, is mentioned with its body hair. But two other functions are added: the six *fu*, which are all the passageways for the food inside the body from ingestion to elimination, and the one hundred joints for all the movements of the body.

Here in the ninth month with the skin and body hair and with the six *fu* and the one hundred joints, all kinds of exchange are possible. We have not only the physical form but also all the movement and circulation. What is complete is not only the skin and joints and so on, but also all the exchanges between the interior and exterior, or all the possibilities of exchange between them which are necessary for the baby to be born and to live. One of the points here is to make us understand the skin has a place as an interface and passageway, and the six *fu* are also a passage. This baby, as soon as it is born, will have to breathe and eat. Everything is ready for that and this is the reason why it says: 'all is complete'.

The reason she 'drinks tasty drinks' is that the woman has to drink something like sweet alcohol, or maybe just water. It is not precise in the text. The problem is that whatever she drinks must be tasty with a subtle richness and she must be happy to drink it. To eat sweet things is along the same lines, but nothing too sweet. Sweet is the harmonization of all the tastes. Some texts also say the danger in wealthy families is that the woman may eat too much sweet, rich food, and this may cause some difficulties in the delivery.

'This is called supporting the body hair and head hair to increase talent and strength.'

This is really to support what is now pushing towards the exterior. The character which is here translated as 'talent' is the same as we saw in the first month, *cai* (才). Now everything is moving outside and the hair is growing and there is an increase in the strength and all the natural endowment. The 'talent' which was potential at the beginning is now expressed in a body complete with its organization and ready to be developed soon by the new little human being.

The *shao yin* of the foot supports all of this, and it is very interesting that the kidneys now arrive at the very end, closing the cycle as we did with the stone. Of course we could say that the kidneys are the origin, but they are at the starting place of the origin which is really a mystery. The kidneys are linked to the origin of the *qi*, the fire, the essences, the *ren* and *du mai*, but when they appear themselves they appear at a different level. For instance, the first month of the pregnancy is dominated by the liver, not the kidneys. The kidneys are linked with the mystery of the origin and the oneness, but their appearance at the end of the process reflects the continuity of the progressive development of life from its hidden, mysterious origin to its complete achievement. So here in the ninth month are the essences of stone, the kidneys and the kidneys meridian, not linked to the specific development or completion of something, but linked to the continuity and the duration, and to the unceasing and perpetual flowing of life. The kidneys ensure the continuity of life from the very beginning to the full accomplishment of the fetus, but they also continue to work throughout the person's life until the very end. It is always from the origin that continuity is ensured.

The link to the vital circulation (*mai* 脈) is interesting if we come back to the character itself. On the left side is the flesh radical (月) and on the right side the part which is explained traditionally as the unceasing flowing of waterways, giving the idea of a continuous flowing and perpetuity. In a human body the *mai* are the continuous circulations of blood and *qi* which make our health. Of course the duration of a life has something to do with the kidneys and the origin which we can call *ming men* (命 門), and the quality of that first impulse decides a person's nature and constitution. It is also interesting to look at the nine months of pregnancy and see how even what is given at the very beginning of life has to be developed, educated and directed in order to result in a good human being. How to eat, how to sit and how to behave during those nine or ten months of pregnancy are detailed in order to allow the full development of all the natural endowment of the baby. This enables a pattern of life for the child which is as perfect as possible in order to ensure the continuity of their vitality.

'In the ninth month, the continuity of vital circulations is completely finished.'

This is a way of saying that in the ninth month all the network of meridians and *luo* (絡), and all the various circulations of blood and *qi* are in exactly the right place with the right movement just waiting to begin working properly. That will occur at birth when food will enter the stomach and the blood and *qi* of the child itself will start to flow through their own network of vital circulations. This is exactly what we have already seen in Lingshu chapter 10:

'The layers of the skin are firm and the body and head hair grow in length. As the grains enter the stomach, the ways of circulation (*mai dao* 脈 道) establish free communication, and blood and *qi* then circulate.'

TENTH MONTH

'In the tenth month of pregnancy the five *zang* are perfectly formed, the six *fu* all communicate, the *qi* of heaven and earth are introduced (*na* 納) into the cinnabar field (*dan tian* 丹 田), which means that the articulations and relays (*guan jie* 關 節) and the spirits of man (*ren shen* 人 神) are all complete.'

This is interesting because now we have a pregnancy with a real human being. At the end of the process the five *zang*, which are also the five elements and the five expressions of the spirit which constitute an individual, are perfectly formed. If they are perfectly formed they are the root of all behaviour and consciousness, of all physiology and psychology. So the six *fu* all communicate, which is what it is important for *fu* to do.

'The *qi* of heaven and earth are introduced into the cinnabar field.'

I will not discuss here what exactly the cinnabar field is. I will just say that it is a place where the *qi* work on the essences in order to maintain life and to produce the best of life. The *qi* move inside and work on the essences to refine them in such a way that the best of human life is produced.

Through its birth the child will take in the *qi* of heaven and earth to breathe and eat, and will warm its essences and *qi* by itself. Before this time the mother had always necessarily been the intermediary, but now there is the potential for this child to become an individual being. To be a human being is not only a matter of breathing and eating, it is to be able to inhale the *qi* of heaven and earth into the cinnabar field. It is the responsibility of each human being to sustain the work of their own essences and *qi*. As we already saw in Guanzi chapter 39, when a baby is born it is able to see, but what a human being can see is not limited to just what is front of their eyes.

The 'articulations and relays' mean all the visible and invisible articulations or joints in the movement of the physical and energetic body.

'The spirits of man, *ren shen* (人 神), are all complete.'

To say this does not mean that they are all present yet, but there is a completeness of the potential of their presence. Some are there, but they will increase with time. The final line of the text is:

'These are the rules for preventing accidents in pregnancy.'

By knowing the phases of the development of the embryo and fetus, and which *qi*, elements and meridians are at work, the mother knows how to behave in order to complement these movements and to prevent miscarriage or disturbance in the fetus. She also knows how to avoid problems for herself during pregnancy, delivery and afterwards.

SUMMARY

The concept of the five elements starting in the fourth month and finishing with the essences of stone in the ninth month is a very ancient idea. We find it in the Mawangdui manuscript which originates from the end of the 3rd century or beginning of the 2nd century BCE. The Huainanzi chapter 7 is also from that time. However, the Mawangdui manuscript does not mention the meridians, although the meridians and the order of their succession do not vary in the medical texts. We find exactly the same thing in the Zhubing Yuanhou Lun as in Sun Simiao and in many other texts. Nobody knows when exactly this started, but certainly the ideas existed before the Zhubing Yuanhou Lun.

There are two cycles: the succession of the elements and the sequence of the seasons. The meridians are always in a *biao li* (表 裏) relationship, but starting with the *yin*, which is a difference from the presentation of the heavenly stems. When we deal with the ten heavenly stems we always start with the *yang*. We saw previously the reason why we have to start with the liver, because we cannot start if nothing has appeared. So it is not the very first beginning, it is the beginning of the appearance of something, however small. The process has already started.

A second point to make is that for this series of the elements the order of appearance is that of the *ke* (剋) cycle, the control cycle. This is because through the *ke* cycle there is an evolution and a change which makes the progress in something. There is not only the succession, there are all the mutations leading to the completed form and organism. However, I think the real reason for the *ke* cycle here is historical. The control cycle was the first cycle to appear which concerned the five elements. There was already a succession in the image of the four seasons, but that did not apply to the five elements as such before the 2nd or 1st centuries BCE. But the control cycle had appeared prior to this in the 3rd century BCE, so it is more ancient.

The expression of the alternation of the five elements was therefore first made through this order of *ke* cycle succession. If we are looking at a text which is quite old, with the correspondences between the fourth and fifth months of the pregnancy and these elements, the only order of alternation was this one of the *ke* cycle. Secondly, this order of succession would also explain why there is the strange association of the wood linked to the bones, the earth to the layers of skin and so on. As we saw earlier with reference to the Huainanzi and the Guanzi, the five element correspondences, and more specifically the medical correspondences, were not fixed at that time. So what we have here in the Zhubing Yuanhou Lun is a series of associations which were made somewhere, at some time, in some schools, and were fixed as a kind of tradition because the text had that practical effect. In fact we find such associations in the Guanzi. For instance in Guanzi chapter 40, blood is associated with water, *qi* with fire, bones with wood and nails with metal. You can also find in chapter 5 of the Suwen a correlation between blood and water, *qi* and fire. This is just to say that there are many variations in the building of a cosmology or a theory.

In these texts, the Zhubing Yuanhou Lun, the Mawangdui manuscript and Sun Simiao, it is possible to divide the ten months into several groups. The first three form a definite series because they are the beginning of something. They describe the creation of a form, or the 'rich paste' of an embryo. After that, for all the other months from four to nine, there are different kinds of beginnings described. The fetus acts and receives, so there is always a beginning in each month. But there is also a completion or achievement of something. In the fourth and fifth months it is blood and *qi*, then the muscular forces and the bones in the sixth and seventh. Finally in the eighth and ninth months it is the *cou li* and the skin and body hair.

Question: I am interested in the tenth month because there is a lot written about the ten lunar months with the assumption that a lunar month is twenty eight days. But a lunar month is actually twenty nine and a half days, so it is really 266 days from the moment of conception, and everything is really completed by the end of the ninth month. So the tenth month is not really a full month and the baby is ready before this?

Absolutely. Also this is the reason why there is no meridian associated with the tenth month. In some later texts they add the bladder meridian, *tai yang* of the foot. But I think it is more beautiful as a system without it because it is not real. As is said even in the ninth month, she 'loosens the belt and waits'. Or in Sun Simiao's tenth month he has something like 'she waits for the right moment'. There is just the idea that everything has been completed and what we said at the beginning, that everything is completed and integrated. Being like that all the five *zang* and the spirits are in a state of full potential. The idea is that there is not as much difference between nine and ten as there is between six and seven, for example. There is nothing more in ten than in nine. Ten does not add something to nine, but is the integration of all the elements of life.

The Zhubing Yuanhuo Lun is not concerned in this text with pathology, it is about the development and education of the fetus (*tai jiao* 胎 教). Here 'education' means the bringing of good influences. What we do when we educate a child is to try and allow them to experience the best influences. Developing a fetus is exactly the same thing. It is always a complete process, so that if you act on the flesh, you are also acting on the mind. What determines the way the fetus and later the baby develops bones and movement is also the structure of their mind and their tendencies.

At the end of Suwen chapter 47 there are two pathologies alluding to pregnancy. One is where a new born baby has convulsions. This baby has had no time to experience anything from the exterior or to react to it, therefore the problem must be related to something which happened during the pregnancy. The explanation given is that during her pregnancy the mother had a great fright (*jing* 驚) and this caused a kind of disruption of the *qi* inside her. The text says the *qi* rise without descending again. It is a bad pattern which has been inscribed in the child and the new born baby may live with this pattern all its life.

Via this pathology we can see a lot of things to be avoided. But what is said in the Zhubing Yuanhou Lun is just that the mother must eat well and in a balanced way, with indications of good tastes which help the development during the month. She must be completely calm and balanced in thinking, and move quietly and appropriately for each stage of the fetus's development. The way to breathe, the way to eat, the way to move and think are all indicated.

Question: What significance do the points mentioned each month have?

I think the points are not there as points to be needled but just to give an indication of the meridian. Sometimes this is very obvious, sometimes not. It is simply a way of recognizing the relevant meridian.

Sun Simiao says that the child who is still a fetus is not completely formed, he has not completely achieved his form and his *yin* and *yang* are not yet well separated. *Zang* and *fu* and the bones and joints are not completely achieved, and this is the reason why the mother must pay such attention to what she eats.

Sun Simiao gives several texts on the evolution of the embryo and then the fetus. The following does have some differences from the Zhubing Yuanhou Lun:

'Rules for the support of the newborn (*yang xiao er fa* 養 小 兒 法):
The child in gestation (*er zai tai* 兒 在 胎)

In the first month it is a embryo (*pei* 胚).

In the second month it is a fetus (*tai* 胎).

In the third month there is blood circulation (*xue mai* 血脈).

In the fourth month the bones of the skull are completed (head, skull and bones, *tou lu gu cheng* 頭顱骨成).

In the fifth month it can move (*neng dong* 能動).

In the sixth month the bones are all present (*ju gu* 具骨).

In the seventh month body and head hair appear (*mao fa sheng* 毛髮生).

In the eight month the body is formed (*xing ti cheng* 形體成).

In the ninth month the *qi* of the grains enter the stomach (*gu qi ru wei* 穀氣入胃).

In the tenth month it is born (*sheng* 生).'

Essentially there are very few differences, even if it is not exactly the same presentation. For instance, there is a differentiation between an embryo and a fetus. The embryo, here expressed by the character *pei* (胚), is something which has no form, it is just like plasticene, and the fetus, expressed by the character *tai* (胎), is something which has already started to have a form. If you take plasticene and heat it, it is too liquid to do anything with, it has to be more compact to start to form something.

This text also moves in pairs. First there are the embryo and fetus, then afterwards the blood circulation (third month) and the bones of the skull (fourth month). In another version of the text, Sun Simiao put a completion of the body form at the fourth month, which avoids having the bones presented twice once at the fourth month as the bones of the skull and head, and secondly at the sixth month as the bones themselves. But we can also understand that the bones completed at the sixth month are those allowing the muscular movements which appear at the fifth month, and these movements strengthen the bones of the limbs and back.

When all the blood and the body and the movement in the body are present, then afterwards there is a turning towards the exterior with the hair and body hair. In the eighth month 'the body is formed' and in the ninth month the *qi* from the grains enter the stomach. At this point the stomach of the fetus starts to function and to make the blood circulate itself. This is the same as in Lingshu chapter 10, and it occurs at birth or just before birth. Nevertheless in both cases it always comes from the mother's blood which is transformed into the milk making the nourishment for the new born baby.

Some variations are found for the eighth month, for example instead of saying that the body is completely formed, this other text says that all the organs, *zang* and *fu*, are fully completed. The meaning is the same, since the body cannot be completed and maintained if the organs are not. For the tenth month it adds: 'the one hundred spirits are completely ready', to indicate that a human being may start to fulfil its destiny.

The end of Sun Simiao's text shows that once the baby is born the process is still not completed, there is a continuation of something. All the potential is present but not yet expressed or realised. Little by little the baby develops and manifests all the potential which is perfected in the five *zang*, the spirits, the six *fu*, the bones and joints and skin and so on.

'Once born, at the end of 60 days (two months) the pupils (*tong zi* 瞳子) are complete (*cheng* 成), [the child] is capable of smiling and of responding to others (*yan xiao ying he ren* 嗲笑應和人).'

Here again is the idea of achieving or completing something. The baby is born but is not completely achieved. So now the baby has to develop according to its own individual nature and circumstances. To be able to smile and respond to another person is something profoundly human and is the reason why the father, in a rich family of course, in the third month after birth will take the baby into his arms, see the baby looking at him and smiling and by analysing all that will name his child. This process is described in the Book of Rites for a noble family. It is at around two to three months that the baby responds to others and starts to focus on them and not just smile at the angels! So it is described at two months in Sun Simiao because he actually observed babies, and at three months in the Book of Rites because of the symbolic value of the number three.

'At the end of 100 days (three and a half months), the *ren mai* appears (*ren mai sheng* 任 脈 生), and [the baby] can turn over and turn back (*fan fu* 反 覆). At the end of 180 days (six months), the bones of the sacrum are complete (*kao gu cheng* 尻 骨 成) and it can sit up on its own (hold itself up sitting). At the end of 210 days (seven months), the bones of the palm (*zhang* 掌) are complete and it can crawl. At the end of 300 days (ten months), the bones of the patella are complete and it can stand up (lean on the ground, *yi di* 倚 地). At the end of 360 days (twelve months), the bones of the knee are complete and it can walk (*xing* 行). If these stages are not respected in their time there is an imbalance somewhere.'

If some development is late, for instance if the baby cannot sit up after six months, or does not start to walk after one year, it is the sign of a weakness or imbalance.

Question: Can you explain how the ren mai appears at 100 days?

This does not mean that the *ren mai* did not exist before hand along with the other meridians. All the *mai* are complete in a way. The mention at this time is really linked with the position of the stomach and the time when the baby is more and more able to eat and digest everything and not just the mother's milk. All essences can be processed directly and the strength which exists between the *ren* and *du mai* means the child is able to move from one side to another by itself. This is the external appearance of the internal possibility of movement.

As we know from Suwen chapter 1 there is another kind of completion of the *ren* and *chong mai* for a woman at two times seven years:

> 'At two times seven years fertility arrives, *ren mai* functions fully while the powerful *chong mai* rises in power. The menses flow downwards in their time and she has children.'

When a woman is pregnant the *ren* and *chong mai* start something new, but they have always had the potential to do so.

THE QIPOLUN 耆婆論

The Qipolun (耆婆論) translates word for word as 'the treatise of old men and women': *qi* (耆) is for old men, *po* (婆) is for old women and *lun* (論) means treatise. 'Old men and old women (*qi po*)' is also the way to transcribe in Chinese the name of the Indian god of longevity, Jiva. In the bibliography written during the Song Dynasty (10-12th century CE), we find several medical treatises under the protection of Jiva. There is a Buddhist undertone in the Qipolun, and it is definitely from the

Song Dynasty. However, it is a text written from another perspective because there are no meridians or elements mentioned, only descriptions of different stages in the development of life.

'In the first month it is like a pearl of dew (*zhu lu* 珠露). In the second month it is like a peach flower (*tao hua* 桃花). In the third month boy and girl are differentiated (*fen* 分). In the fourth month the bodily appearance is complete (*xing xiang ju* 形象具). In the fifth month the musculature and bones are complete (*jin gu cheng* 筋骨成). In the sixth month body and head hair appear (*mao fa sheng* 毛髮生). In the seventh month, by the journey of its *hun* (*you qi hun* 遊其魂), the child can move its left hand. In the eight month, by the journey of its *po* (*you qi po* 遊其魄), the child can move its right hand. In the ninth month the body turns three times (makes three turns, *san zhuan shen* 三轉身). In the tenth month, it receives the *qi* in sufficiency (*shou qi zu* 受氣足).'

This is a beautiful presentation, but completely different from the texts we have been looking at. The 'pearl of dew' is something which is very important because it is essences which are almost *qi* and *qi* which are almost essences. It is something which looks like a pearl in form but which is very light and impossible to actually touch. You do not know if it is liquid or air. It is the best of the *jing qi* (精氣) because it is the most subtle expression of the alliance of essences and *qi*. This is why the immortals feed on this white dew or pearl of dew. Perhaps its appearance here is to represent the most subtle thing coming from a man in the form of his semen? So it stands for the most subtle aspect of the *qi* of the father and the essences of the mother. There is something very moving in the fragility of this beginning.

As we saw in the Huainanzi during the second month there was a bulge, and this is exactly the same thing. The peach flower here evokes the spring, just as the dew evokes the early morning. We are somewhere in the realm of the liver and gallbladder if you like, but this is not a correspondence as such. It is more a resonance with the beginning of something, of a day, or a year. Perhaps there is something to do with the form of the embryo at this time? But even without these associations we can still have a symbolic level of interpretation, and still with this sense of poetic fragility.

In the third month there is a form because there is sexual differentiation. After that, in the fourth month, there is the bodily appearance of something. The three first months are therefore the period of budding and blossoming. The form of the fourth month combines with the muscular forces and bones in the fifth month, and the body and head hair in the sixth month. Months four, five and six are for the formation of all the body and we can say that they are the work of the earth. Four is the appropriate number for form, and the correct place to start the work of earth in giving shape.

In the seventh and eighth months the *hun* (魂) and *po* (魄) appear. In other texts the *po* may come first and the *hun* afterwards, or they may come at different times during gestation. We are now at a stage when the realisation of the human being with a soul is expressed by the *hun* and *po* and all the movement of life which they command. Perhaps in the ninth month this movement is expressed in the body by turning three times? Three is the number of *qi*. I do not know if the fetus really does move the left hand before the right in these months, but I think the important thing is that we have the *hun* first and then the *po*, in the likeness of heaven and earth. They come together but one comes first! The specific nature of a human being has now arrived. If the potential of essences and *qi* have a form, then the spiritual animation of the *hun* and *po* must be present.

In the tenth month 'it receives the *qi* in sufficiency'. Everything which makes the *qi* and all their movement is complete. The baby is male or female, so there is a specific balance of blood and *qi*, and all the bodily form and the spiritual animation are complete. If you consider the first three months you could say that they represent heaven, earth and mankind, because at the beginning the pearl of dew is something suspended between heaven and earth, the peach flower is the blossoming on earth, and then the differentiation between boy and girl is the level of the human being.

THE LUXINJING 顱 囟 經

The Luxinjing, The Book of the Skull, is a text from around the same period. It is found in Zhang Jiebin (1563-1640) who said that this book belonged to a school of shamans. It is a very interesting text.

'In the first month the embryo is in the uterus (*tai bao* 胎 胞) and essences and blood (*jing xue* 精 血) condense (coagulate, *ning* 凝).

In the second month the embryo takes form (*tai xing* 胎 形) and begins to constitute a fetus (*pei* 胚).

In the third month the *yang* spirits (*yang shen* 陽 神) make (*wei* 為) the three *hun*.

In the fourth month the *yin* spiritual influences (*yin ling* 陰 靈) make the seven *po*.

In the fifth month the five elements distinguish (are divided into, *fen* 分) five *zang*.

In the sixth month the six musical pipes (*liu lu* 六 律) fix (determine, *ding* 定) the six *fu*.

In the seventh month the essences open the orifices (*jing kai qiao* 精 開 竅), and the light circulates (*tong guang ming* 通 光 明).

In the eight month the original spirits (*yuan shen* 元 神) are all present (*ju* 具), they make the authentic spiritual influences descend (*jiang zhen ling* 降 真 靈).

In the ninth month the tissue that envelops the residence (*gong shi luo bu* 宮 室 羅 布) is well fixed

(determined, *ding* 定) and gives birth to a human
being (*sheng ren* 生人).
In the tenth month it receives the *qi* in sufficiency
(*shou qi zu* 受氣足) and the ten thousand images
are perfectly complete (*wan xiang cheng* 萬象
成).'

Here the first division is obviously by pairs, one and
two, three and four and so on. First comes *tai* (胎) and
afterwards *pei* (胚), which is the opposite order from
that found in other texts. But this is not very important
for the meaning.

'In the first month the embryo is in the uterus (*tai
bao* 胎胞) and essences and blood (*jing xue* 精血)
condense (coagulate, *ning* 凝).'

Here the 'embryo' has to be understood not as an
embryo itself but as the possibility of having a child.
The character *tai* (胎) is used, particularly in later
books, for everything which is the process of pregnancy.
The meaning is therefore that in the first month the
process of pregnancy starts in the uterus by means of a
condensation of essences and blood.

The essences and blood obviously stand here for
what comes from the father and mother. The essences
are the same character as sperm, *jing* (精), so there is
the condensation and coagulation of the essences from
both parents: sperm from the man and blood from the
woman. This is a very normal way to look at this process

in a treatise of this period. It is exactly the same idea as we have seen before, the process of condensation and coming together, with the unity of the two essences coming from the parents. In the second month the process of making of a new life takes on more and more real form and it is possible then to speak of a fetus. It is now not only something which is a potential of the parents' essences, it is a unique new life on its own way. This is the constitution, and the beginning of a new being.

Immediately after this beginning comes spiritual animation, or the potential for the spirits to be present. If the essences are pure and clear enough, and are able to make a human body, then they are also capable of attracting the spirits of heaven. The same idea is expressed in Huainanzi chapter 7 where the subtle and essential *qi* are said to form human beings and the unclear, coarse *qi* form animals. These are not the same essences. If human essences are able to coagulate and constitute the beginning of a new life, then the result will be that the spirits of heaven are attracted and will come to dwell in that human body. The pairing of essences and spirits is the building of the *jing shen* (精 神), the vital spirits of mankind. A person maintains the best of their vital spirits as long as they are able to renew their human essences in their quality and richness, and not disturb and deplete them through emotions, exhaustion, diet and so on.

Nowadays people are often too fixated on knowing exactly when a certain process or stage is achieved in a pregnancy, for example at what moment the *hun* enter. It is impossible to answer those questions. You will always find another text telling you something different. These things are not specific moments in time but a continuous, unfolding process. As soon as there are human essences and something starts to make a human form, then spirits will be attracted. Because they are attracted then the movement of *qi* inside that life will be made in the likeness of what we call *hun*. It will be a model of attraction to heaven, which is a definition of the *hun*. The *yang* spirits make appear, or are, the three *hun*.

Are the spirits *yin* or *yang*? The answer is that they are behind *yin* and *yang*. At that time in Chinese history the *shen* (神) could be taken in a couple with *ling* (靈), and therefore it is possible to place *shen* on the *yang* side and *ling* on the *yin* side. However, this can only be done within this couple, and only after a certain date. Before the daoist texts of the 9th and 10th centuries CE it is not possible to find this as such.

It is impossible to explain everything which lies behind *shen* and *ling* because it is very complex. From the text of The Book of the Skull we can simply know that the *shen* are on the side of heaven, have a movement of initiation and can start the process, while *ling* are on the side of the development or fruition of the initiating action of the *shen*. So the *shen* are the spirits and the *ling* are the spiritual influences or impulses. The pattern for *ling* (靈) is found in the rain (雨). The rain descends from heaven because the shamanesses depicted at the bottom of the character (*wu* 巫) are dancing and praying with their mouths wide open. The mouth wide open is represented by three mouths (*kou* 口). The rain which comes will allow the crops to ripen, give fertility to the soil, and bring beneficial effects to life. There is an useful quality in *ling* which we see in the image of the rain. Rain means no starvation!

Ling is easily linked with the *po* (魄) which are connected to the essences and earth, and to life which follows not leads. The *hun* (魂) take the lead. It is a question of precedence again. This is interesting because we have heaven and earth within our self. They are not only present in the essences of the embryo or fetus, but also in everything which makes the depth of all human life by the *shen ling* and the *hun* and *po*. The *shen* produce the possibility and efficacy of the three *hun*, and the *ling* produce the *yin po*.

In the fifth and sixth months there is another couple comprised of the five elements and the six musical pipes, linking up with the five *zang* and the six *fu*. The five elements are divided into five *zang* so that each element is on its own and is able to reproduce itself in the fetus as one of the five *zang*. What is less easy to understand is the relationship between the six *fu* and the six musical pipes. If the five *zang* are the five elements, they are operating at the level of five, and therefore the five notes. The five notes are the way to classify sound, but the six pipes are the device by which those sounds are produced. To play music you have to have notes, but you also have to have pipes through which the air is sent in order to play those notes. The result is a specific sound which is neither a note nor a pipe.

The five *zang* or five *qi* are in the likeness of the five elements or the five notes. Here they represent everything which encompasses and organizes life. The six *fu*, being in the likeness of the six musical pipes, are the physical pipes or tubes which allow us to resonate in the detail. This means that here the six *fu* represent a physical tube through which the essences pass and which allow the five *zang* to express in detail the functioning of the human body and the five *qi*. In short, by the passage through the six *fu*, the clear is assimilated and the turbid rejected. Then the essences allow the functioning of the five *zang*.

This is something which we find regularly in texts, and it is always difficult for us to understand why the five *zang* are the same thing as the five notes, and why the six *fu* are the same thing as the six musical pipes. Yes they are five and six, but the real explanation is a bit more involved. Five is for the control of the various movements of *qi* and six is for sustaining the expression. Without the *fu* there is no integration and assimilation of the essences which nourish the five *zang*. This is the vision. The *fu* of the digestive tract are like tubes.

In the seventh month 'the essences open the orifices (*jing kai qiao* 精 開 竅), and the light circulates (*tong guang ming* 通 光 明).' *Kai qiao* (開 竅) is used in many classical texts meaning to open the orifice. For example in Suwen chapter 4 it says the liver opens its orifice at the eye, and the spleen opens its orifice at the mouth, and so on. The characters describe the link between a *zang* and its orifice. A very ancient idea, also found in Huainanzi chapter 4, is that the condensation of *qi* forms the essences. This allows us to live and allows each of the *zang* to function freely.

When it says 'the light circulates' it means communicates. The character *tong* (通) is also widely used for the connection between the organ and its orifice. The liver communicates with the eyes, the spleen communicates with the mouth, and so on. For *guang ming* (光 明) this kind of circulation is also an enlightenment. At the level of the upper orifices, which are also the sense organs, there needs to be not only good communication of essences, but also the spiritual enlightenment coming from the *zang*. The five *zang* are the spiritual power, so the eyes not only see but also have discernment about what is seen. The same thing is true for the other upper orifices. You can see this in Lingshu chapter 17. More than this, the upper orifices are considered, in Huainanzi chapter 7 for instance, as the passage for the vital spirits:

'Openings and orifices are windows and doors of the vital spirits.'

At the highest level therefore these upper orifices are taken as all the passages for the vital spirits, or the life which comes from the innermost part. In this way the character *qiao* (竅) itself, meaning orifice, is something which is explained as a spreading out of life. The upper part is a cave or hollow inside the earth (穴), an opening in the earth as a cavern or grotto. It is also the character translated as an acupuncture point. The lower part may be analyzed as a releasing (放) of light (白), to let the light go out. According to traditional etymology therefore an orifice is a hollow through which light is emitted.

Through this text, which focuses on the spiritual power, we have the building of the sense organs and their relationship with the *zang* and with their good use at all levels within a human being.

For the eighth month it says:

'The original spirits (*yuan shen* 元 神) are all present (*ju* 具), they make the authentic spiritual influences descend (*jiang zhen ling* 降真靈).'

The 'original spirits' are the spirits which come from the origin, or the spirits which are here due to the quality of the original essences, the original *qi* and nature of the being. Do not forget that the brain is sometimes called the *fu* of the *yuan shen* (元 神), the spirits linked with the origin. The spirits come to the original nature, and this is the reason why the brain is linked to the kidneys. I think by practice and through the process of life a person is able to attract a myriad of spirits, and to be at one with the spiritual power. But this passage is a way of saying that within each human being there is naturally enough spiritual presence to be fully human. After that it is up to the person themself to cultivate the ability to be at one with the spirits or not.

Since the spirits constitute the natural and celestial life in a person, the spiritual influences are attracted and descend. If someone is in the appropriate and proper place in their life it means that everything is going according to the heavenly impulse, and in that case the result will be complete power and efficiency of life.

'In the ninth month the tissue that envelops the residence (*gong shi luo bu* 宮室羅布) is well fixed (determined, *ding* 定) and gives birth to a human being (*sheng ren* 生人).'

This is the end of the formation of the human being with the limit of their body fixed at the level of the skin, but the skin is not mentioned here because this is not a medical text. There is a sort of web around us which acts as the limit of our being, and which at the ninth month is completely achieved. This is finally a full human being.

'In the tenth month it receives the *qi* in sufficiency (*shou qi zu* 受氣足) and the ten thousand images are perfectly complete (*wan xiang cheng* 萬象成).'

This is the same *xiang* (象) as was seen in the third month of the Zhubing Yuanhou Lun. All the attributes of the human being, everything which composes a human life, are now perfectly accomplished and ready to be expressed.

Question: Why in the tenth month does it say the ten thousand images?

In a human being, the ten thousand images are in the likeness of the ten thousand beings in the universe, between heaven and earth; so that the human being is the perfect mirror of heaven and earth and the human body is able to correspond completely and perfectly to the work of heaven and earth. Every detail is perfect and in unity. This is the pattern which is active, and which actively forms what we may become. The period of gestation enables a new human being to become a mirror of the intertwining of heaven and earth:

'Mankind is the combined virtue of heaven and earth, the interaction of *yin* and *yang*, the union of earthly and heavenly spirits, and the best from the *qi* of the five elements. ... Therefore mankind is the heart of heaven and earth, and the perfect embodiment of the five elements.' (Liji, Liyun. Translation based on Legge)

APPENDIX

TABLE OF CORRESPONDENCES FROM THE ZHUBING YUANHOU LUN

MONTH	IN THE FETUS	FORM	MOTHER'S MERIDIAN	MASTERS
FIRST	Beginning of form	Innate material	Foot jue yin - Liv	Blood
SECOND	Beginning of rich paste	Beginning of storing	Foot shao yang - Gb	Essences
THIRD	Beginning of fetus	To change according to outside images	Hand jue yin - HM (P)	Vital spirits
FOURTH	Water	Blood circulation	Hand shao yang - TH	Six fu
FIFTH	Fire	Qi	Foot tai yin - Sp	Four limbs
SIXTH	Metal	Musculature/movement	Foot yang ming - St	Mouth and eyes
SEVENTH	Wood	Bones	Hand tai yin - Lu	Skin and body hair
EIGHTH	Earth	Layers of the skin	Hand yang ming - LI	Nine orifices
NINTH	Stone	Skin and body hair, the six fu, the 100 joints	Foot shao yin - Ki	Vital circulation

INDEX

INDEX

ENGLISH LANGUAGE BOOK REFERENCES

Donald Harper: *Early Chinese Medical Literature, The Mawangdui Medical Manuscripts,* Kegan Paul International, London and New York, 1998

Legge : *The Sacred Books of China*

W. Allyn Ricketts, *Guanzi, Political, Economic, and Philosophical Essays from Early China,* Princeton Library of Asian Translations, Princeton University Press, New Jersey, USA, 1998

Burton Watson, *The Complete Works of Chuang Tzu,* Columbia University Press, USA, 1968